this period in my life

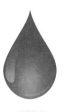

A period guide book and journal

SASKIA BOUJO

First published in Great Britain 2020

Copyright © 2020 Saskia Boujo

ISBN: 978-1-5272-6293-5

A catalogue record for this book is available from the British Library

For more information visit www.saskiaboujo.com

Printed and bound in Great Britain by Pensord Press
www.pensord.co.uk

**THIS BOOK IS DEDICATED TO MY GIRLS ELISE, UMA AND LUCILLE
AND GOD DAUGHTER ISAMOO**

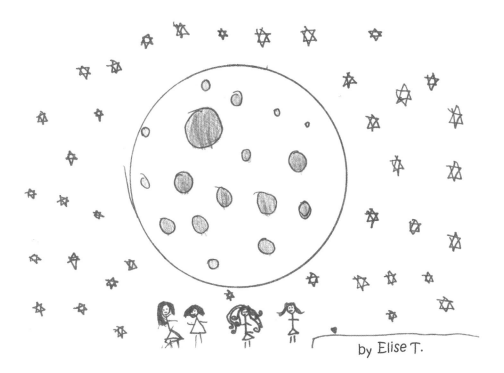

by Elise T.

AND TO ALL THOSE WHO MENSTRUATE

What people are saying about 'this period in my life'

"I wish this book had existed when I was growing up and knew precisely nothing about my anatomy or how periods work. Knowledge is power and this book is stuffed full of the good stuff."

Emma Barnett, journalist and broadcaster, and author of 'Period. About Bloody Time'

"So far as I know...there is no such book with such simple facts and images... it's a wonderful contribution for young people, for families in general - plain speaking...direct...no nonsense.
It is a book we should all have had as children.
It's a beautiful contribution to human life!"

Jon Snow, journalist and broadcaster

"I wish I had had this excellent book when I had my first period. It was such a confusing time and the information was so sketchy. Saskia Boujo talks about periods in such a straightforward - even funny - way. She debunks all of the inaccurate stories that are told, and totally removes any sense of fear someone might have. I particularly appreciated her discussion of period poverty and her good suggestions about what can be done. An essential guide for any young person approaching puberty."

Rosie Boycott, writer and editor

"A powerful book designed to spread period confidence and combat period stigma, which holds us all back! Such a helpful read to any one of any age and gender."

Laura Coryton, 'End Tampon Tax' petition starter and co-founder of 'Sex Ed Matters'

"Makes me wish I had periods too!"

Earl of Uxbridge

DISCLAIMER

Please keep in mind that all opinions expressed in this book are solely my own. While I have experience as a fellow menstruator and as an educator - and listening to the views of young people for many years - I am not a medic, expert physician, nutritionist or registered dietician. The information in this book is intended as advice and may not be used as a substitute for professional advice and/or information, as circumstances will vary from person to person. Use at your own risk.

The publication is written and published to provide accurate information relevant to the subject matter presented. Care has been taken to confirm the accuracy of the information given, and describe generally accepted practices. However, the author, editor, and publisher are not responsible for errors or omissions.

LET'S TRANSLATE ALL THAT!

Let's translate all that! Essentially, this book is a guide only and should not replace the advice of any trusted adult or professional. Before you consider taking any medication, trying out PMS remedies, changing your diet, attempting new exercise or experimenting with new menstrual products, SPEAK TO YOUR TRUSTED ADULT!

CONTENTS

SECTION 2: TUNING INTO YOUR CYCLE

SECTION 3: BONUS CONTENT

SECTION 4: REFERENCE

Know
yourself

INTRODUCTION

Blood.

What's it all about?

This book is written and designed for every person who bleeds once a month and deserves to fully understand what on earth it all means. The aim is to get to know your body, and yourself, even better.

There are two parts to this book:

> **Section 1** *contains information to help you understand, manage and tune into your menstrual cycle.*

> **Section 2** *has charts and tables for you to plot and track your period, as well as allowing you to write down any physical and emotional symptoms you might be experiencing.*

This is a really special time, a big transition from childhood to adulthood, so...

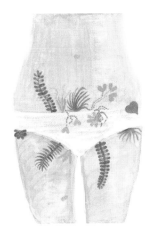

TAKE IT EASY ON YOURSELF

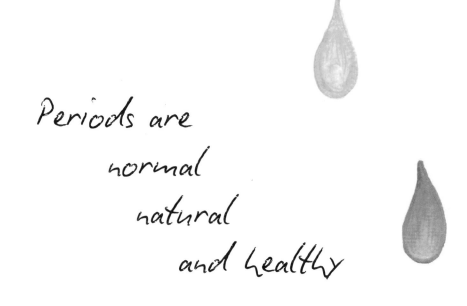

Periods are
normal
natural
and healthy

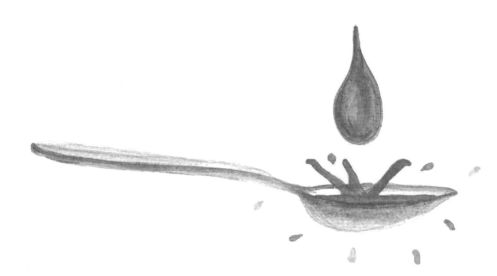

1

PERIOD FACTS

- Periods can start anywhere between the ages of **8 and 15** years old.

- Periods usually last between **4 and 7 days**, and once regular, bleeding happens once a month.

- During a period, approximately **6-8 teaspoons** of blood is lost over the course of 4 to 7 days.

- It can take up to 5 years for your period to be regular, with the average menstrual cycle lasting between **27 and 33 days**.

- Most people who menstruate will have between **400 and 500 periods** in their lifetime.

- There are over **200 million people** in the world menstruating right now.

- The bleeding is the **first** of 4 phases of the menstrual cycle.

- Periods are a sign of fertility, good health and symbolise the start of **adulthood**.

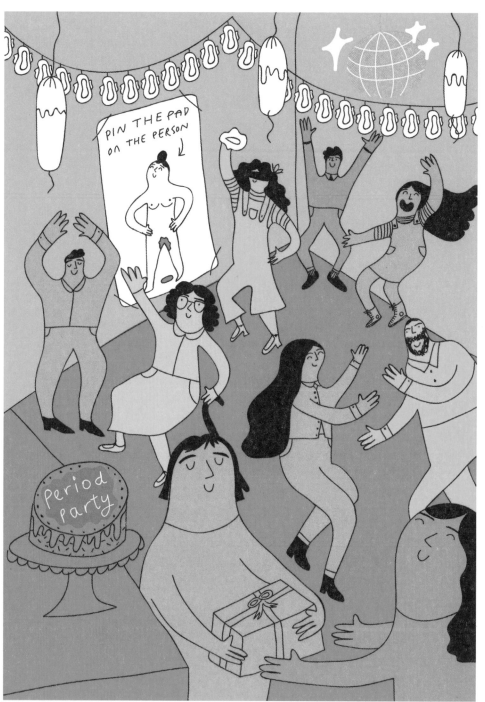

Artwork by Natalie Byrne, 'Period Party', 2020

2

FIRST
PERIOD

Your first period, or first bleed, is known as the **Menarche**. In many cultures this is seen as the start of adulthood and therefore something to celebrate. Here's how some cultures mark the occasion:

- The pigmy tribes of **Africa** sing songs whilst sitting in a circle to mark the start of a young person's journey towards adulthood.
- In **Japan**, red rice is made and eaten to mark this new phase of life.
- In **India**, to celebrate Ambubachi Mela, locals hold a four-day festival to celebrate fertility.
- In some **European cultures**, red gifts are given and a family party is organised to mark the occasion.

How will you celebrate your first period? (no pressure!) ....

....

....

What to expect

From now on you should expect to bleed irregularly for the first few years, as on average it takes about 5 years for the bleeding to occur at roughly the same time every month, or every 28 days. This means that initially you may want to be prepared in case you are caught off guard!

<u>Useful tips to be prepared:</u>

♦ Keep a few menstrual pads or other products in your **school bag**, safely in a small purse. If you lend one to a friend in need, make sure you replace it. It may also be useful to have a spare set of underwear in your bag too, in case you bleed through, as well as a small plastic bag if you are wearing re-usable items.

♦ **At school** find out where the supplies of menstrual products are kept, and tell your friends so they're also aware of where to go. As a student, you are entitled to free donations of menstrual products, so if you feel able to, ask a teacher or school nurse.

♦ Locate your **nearest chemist** or local shop so that you know where to stock up on menstrual products.

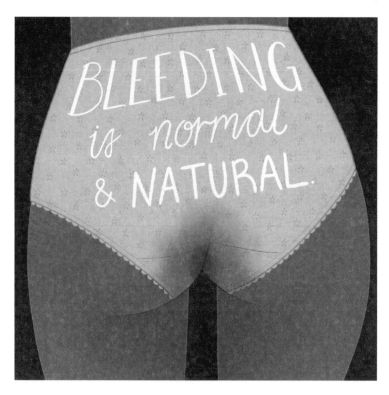

Artwork By Charlotte Willcox 'Bleeding is normal' 2019

3

SCIENTIFIC PERIOD

Your period is one of many signs that you are entering into a new chapter of your life: Adulthood. You may have noticed some other signs that your body is changing, which are all part of adolescence, also known as **puberty**.

The bigger picture
It is highly likely that before you first started bleeding you experienced some other bodily changes that are all normal, healthy and natural parts of puberty. These may include, but are not limited to:

- Discharge in your underwear
- Hair growth under your arms, around your vulva and legs
- Developing breasts
- Generally feeling different!

What is discharge? Discharge is fluid that comes out of your vagina. It helps keep it clean and prevents infection.

All of this is normal, natural and healthy

You can write down here the changes you first observed your body going through, including any thoughts you've had.

1 ....

2 ....

3 ....

4 ....

5 ....

Your period starting is one of the many signs that everything is in working order. So pat yourself on the back for having reached this important milestone in your life!

Well done!

The Vulva

The **vulva** is the whole of the genital area. The vulva has 3 holes, each with their own function:

- The urethra: lets out urine
- The vagina: lets out menstrual blood
- The anus: lets out faeces (poo)

It can be useful to take a look at your vulva (using a small mirror) as **all vulvas are different**. Just as we have different eyes, hair and hands, our vulvas vary in shape, size and colour, and are very rarely completely symmetrical.

Feel free to familiarise yourself with your genital area using a small mirror. The anus and vaginal opening are quite easy to locate but the urethra is a little tricky to find. Have a go! All these holes are protected by labia minora (inner lips) and labia majora (outer lips). This diagram has been drawn without pubic hair to allow for clarity, but usually **it is entirely normal for pubic hair to grow all over the mont pubis,** as well as all around the lips, as its purpose is to provide a layer of protection.

<u>Top to bottom - literally!</u>

Period blood will leave your body through your vagina, but as the holes are all located quite close together, things might feel a little 'messy' down there. One drop of blood will change the colour of your urine, so although it may look like you are weeing blood, rest assured, you're not. Also, when wiping after a poo, it is normal to see blood on the tissue paper.

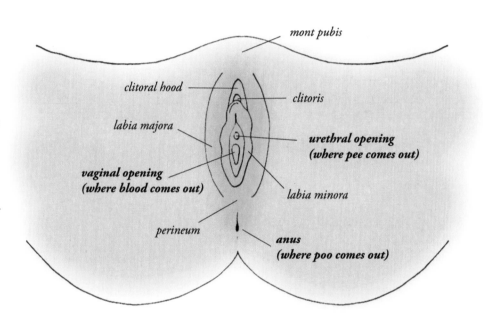

Artwork by Mille Baring, "Vulva", 2020

<u>The inside story</u>

Now that we've explored the external part of your anatomy and the fact that blood leaves your body once a month, let's take a look at what's happening inside.

The start of your period is just one of the signs that your body is preparing to, one day, welcome a baby. Every month one of your ovaries releases an egg that travels down your fallopian tube to reach your uterus (also known as your womb).

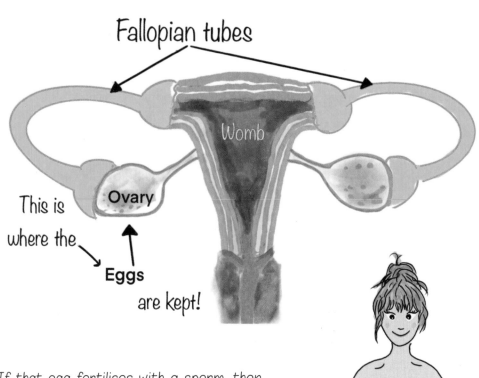

Fallopian tubes

Womb

This is where the

Ovary

Eggs

are kept!

If that egg fertilises with a sperm, then there is a chance that an embryo is created, which could then grow into a baby. The baby would develop inside the womb. In the event that fertilisation does take place, the womb is preparing to welcome it by getting nice and cosy, soft and warm **just in case** an embryo nestles inside there. Getting soft and cosy means that the lining of your womb gets thicker and 'cosier' throughout your cycle for the embryo to snuggle into.

Most months no fertilisation takes place, and therefore that cosy, soft womb serves no purpose, so the lining of the womb falls away. And that falling away is your period.

Simple? errr...NO!

Artwork By Lisa Joly, 2020

Let's try and use some imagery to make this clearer.

A nice analogy is imagining the womb as a nest. This nest is building slowly, layer upon layer, throughout the month in preparation for an egg to settle into it. That way, should an egg settle in here, it may grow and develop and, one day, perhaps become a chick. However, if no egg comes, the nest breaks away, and falls off the tree to the ground. And that 'falling away' of the nest, is your period.

This chain of events repeats every month, which is why it is called a Menstrual 'Cycle'.

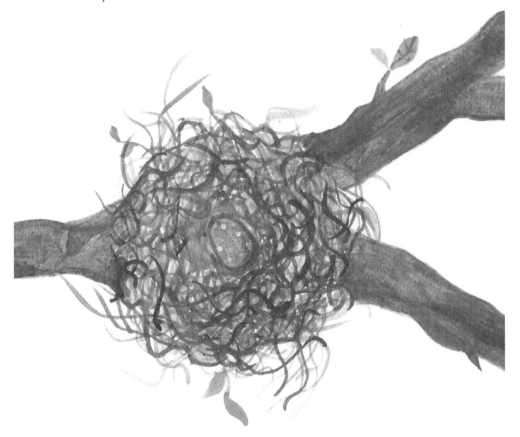

Isn't your body amazing!

Please note:

Starting your first period means that your body is physically able to get pregnant. Although that might be the furthest thing from your mind at this point, how amazing to know you hold the power to CREATE LIFE one day if you so choose!

If you are sexually active, it is important to take precautions and look into contraception if you do not want to get pregnant. Speak to a trusted adult about your options.

ACTIVITY IDEA – A Helping Hand

Draw or trace the outline of your hand in the free pages at the back of the book, or on page 159. Then, write down the name of a **trusted adult** on each finger. One should not be a family member (eg. neighbour, doctor, teacher…).

Having trusted adults in your life is important. They are the people you can turn to when you have a problem, or when you have questions. To find one, make a list of the adults in your life, then decide which of these adults make you feel safe and respected, and **who will listen**.

4

SEASONAL PERIOD

The menstrual cycle moves from one phase to another, repeating the same cycle on average 12 times in one year. Can you think of any other repetitive events, or cycles of life, in nature or around you? Write them down here:

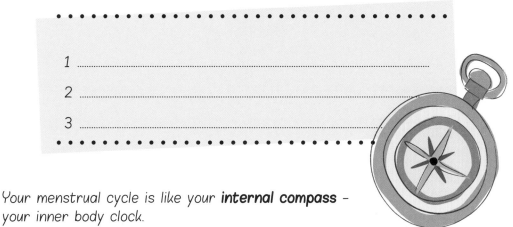

1 ....

2 ....

3 ....

Your menstrual cycle is like your **internal compass** – your inner body clock.

Just like the fact that days end and nights begin, and the sun sets and the moon rises, our menstrual cycles repeat the same 4 phases each month. It's a bit like a clock that goes round and round. There are **4 parts** to the Menstrual Cycle. Bleeding is just the first part (see the diagram on the next page).

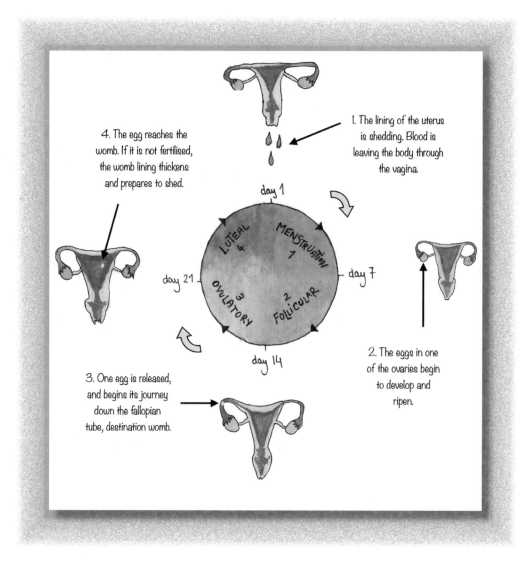

4. The egg reaches the womb. If it is not fertilised, the womb lining thickens and prepares to shed.

1. The lining of the uterus is shedding. Blood is leaving the body through the vagina.

day 1

LUTEAL 4

MENSTRUATION 1

day 21

OVULATORY 3

FOLLICULAR 2

day 7

day 14

2. The eggs in one of the ovaries begin to develop and ripen.

3. One egg is released, and begins its journey down the fallopian tube, destination womb.

Please note that everyone's phases will vary in length. This diagram serves as a guide only.

The 4 Seasons

Think of the entire monthly cycle as a year and each phase as a season. Just as the seasons bring on changes in our environment, such as leaves falling in autumn and flowers growing in spring, your menstrual cycle triggers changes in your body, as well as creating hormones in your body that make you feel different from week to week.

Each phase of the menstrual cycle can be linked to a season, as well as a phase of the moon:

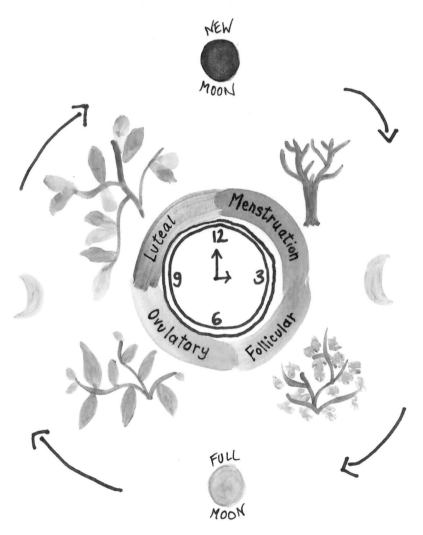

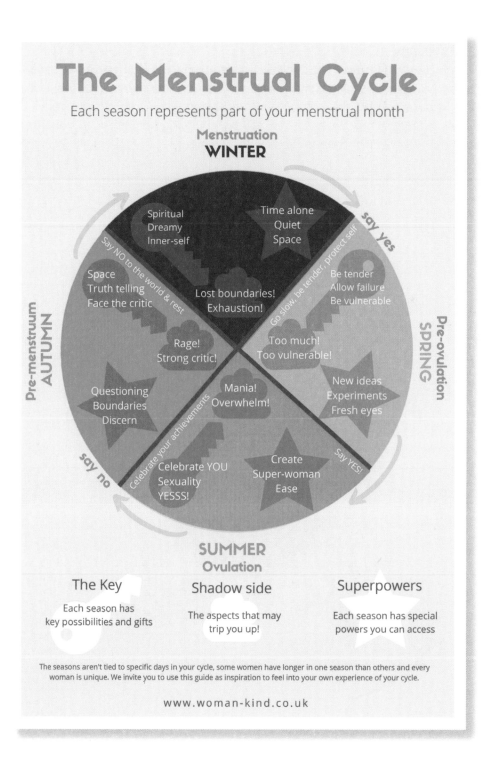

The Menstrual Cycle

Each season represents part of your menstrual month

Menstruation
WINTER

Spiritual
Dreamy
Inner-self

Time alone
Quiet
Space

say yes

Say NO to the world & rest

Go slow, be tender, protect self

Space
Truth telling
Face the critic

Lost boundaries!
Exhaustion!

Be tender
Allow failure
Be vulnerable

Pre-menstruum
AUTUMN

Pre-ovulation
SPRING

Rage!
Strong critic!

Too much!
Too vulnerable!

Questioning
Boundaries
Discern

Mania!
Overwhelm!

New ideas
Experiments
Fresh eyes

Celebrate your achievements

say no

Celebrate YOU
Sexuality
YESSS!

Create
Super-woman
Ease

Say YES!

SUMMER
Ovulation

The Key

Each season has
key possibilities and gifts

Shadow side

The aspects that may
trip you up!

Superpowers

Each season has special
powers you can access

The seasons aren't tied to specific days in your cycle, some women have longer in one season than others and every woman is unique. We invite you to use this guide as inspiration to feel into your own experience of your cycle.

www.woman-kind.co.uk

Chart designed by Kate Codrington & Leora Leboff at Woman kind

Look at the image on the page opposite. For now, just focus on the words on the outside of the circle. Write down in the table below which season is associated with which part of the menstrual cycle:

Colour	Season	Phase
Brown		
	Spring	
		Ovulation
		Pre-menstuation

ACTIVITY IDEA –
Seasonal wheel

1. Draw around the base of a mug
   and cut out the circle.

2. Fold in half, and fold again.
   Unfold and you should have 4 equal parts.

3. Trace lines over the folds.

4. Can you name each
   phase of your cycle?

5. Then decorate with
   matching seasons
   and moons !

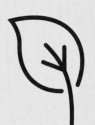
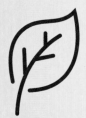

17

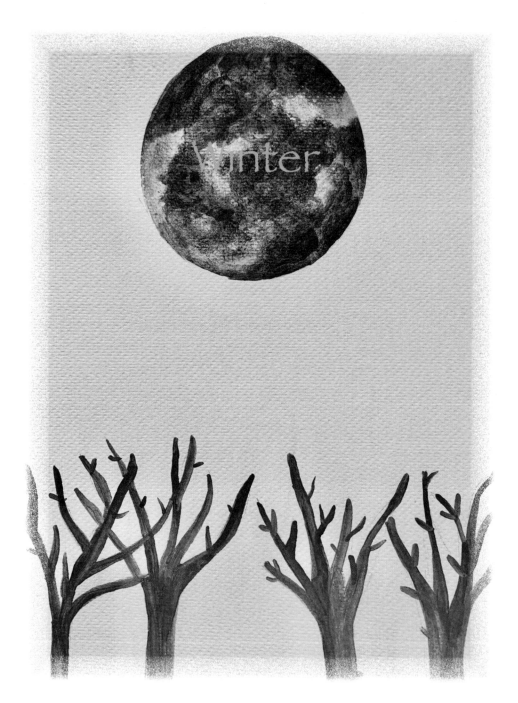

Blood is leaving the body through the vagina

1

Menstruation Phase Care Plan

	Approximate Day: 1-7
Physically	Bloated, fatigued, cramps, backache, sensitive
Mentally	Tired, inward, reflective, intuitive
A great time to...	Set new intentions Write in a journal
You might feel like...	Curling up with a hot water bottle Doing nothing
Try to avoid	Processed, sweet, spicy, snacky food Alcohol, coffee and red meat
At night	Sweats are likely so loose, cotton clothing is best

The egg is ripening in one of the ovaries

2

Follicular Phase Care Plan

The 4 Seasons

	Approximate Day: 7-14
Physically	Energised, vibrant, fresh
Mentally	Focused, confident, creative
A great time to...	Take action Start new creative projects
You might feel like...	Going out. Having fun
Try to avoid	Too much red meat
At night	Unwind before bedtime for a good night's sleep

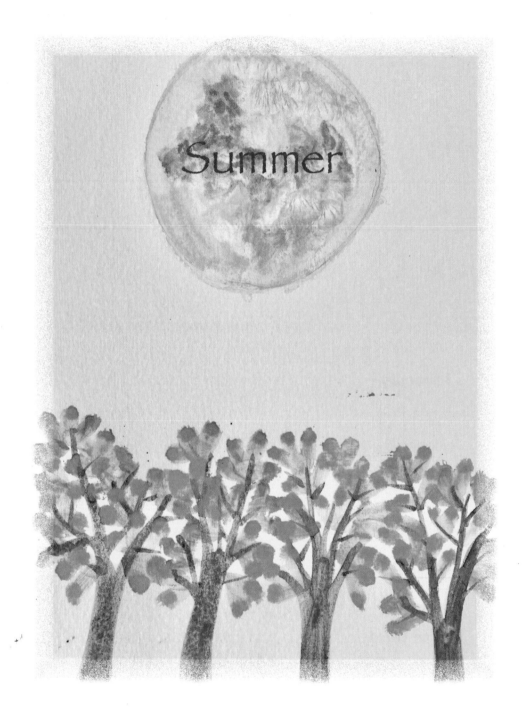

The egg is travelling down the fallopian tube

3

Ovulatory Phase
Care Plan

Let Go

	Approximate Day: 14-21
Physically	Fertile, ripe, free, sexy
Mentally	Sociable, expressive, radiant, confident
A great time to...	Let go! Surrender to what you love
You might feel like...	You relate well or connect better to others
Try to avoid	Too many carbohydrates
At night	Sleep will be deep so get cosy

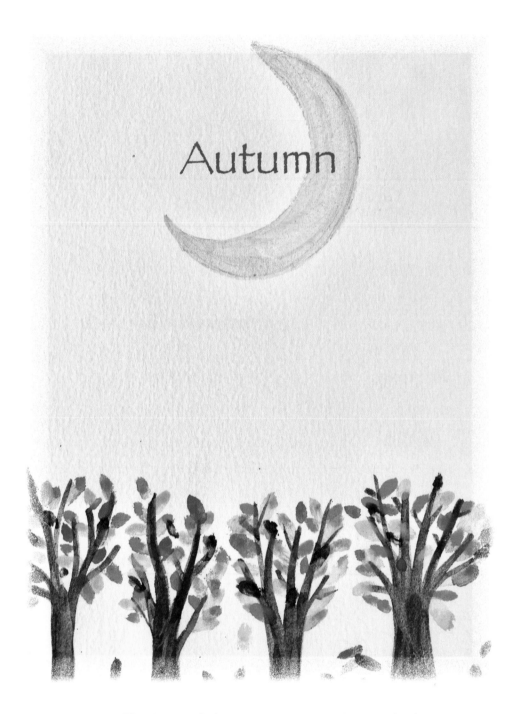

Autumn

The lining of the uterus is preparing to shed

4

Luteal Phase
Care Plan

	Approximate Day: 21-28
Physically	Hungry, bloated, thirsty
Mentally	Sensitive, critical, pensive
A great time to…	Release anything unwanted Be domestic and nest
You might feel like…	Evaluating your desires, needs and fears
Try to avoid	Snacking too much on comfort foods
At night	A change in hormones means your sleep may be interrupted and increasingly so in the run up to your bleed

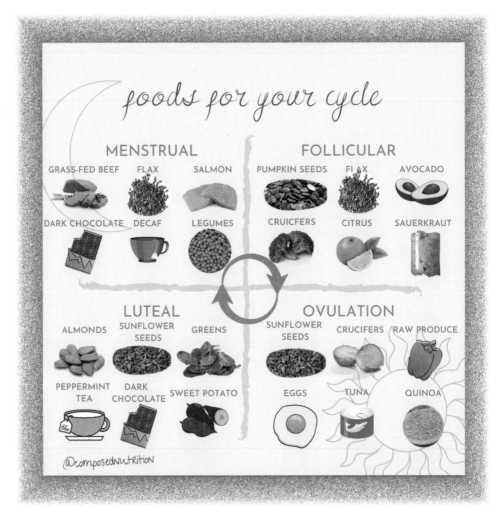

Artwork by Krista King, "Foods for your cycle", 2020

Nourishing each phase

As your body moves through the different phases of your cycle, it might be giving you clues as to what it needs in order to travel as well as possible through each of the 4 phases. Some days you might feel dehydrated and on others you might feel an uncontrollable desire to snack. **Your body is communicating with you about what it needs**, but it's easy to get led down the wrong path, especially when it comes to snacking!

We just had to share Krista King's artwork (left). As your hormones fluctuate throughout the month, certain **foods and nutrients support each phase**. Obviously, it's good to keep a balanced diet at all times, but this image gives you a few easy steps to ensure you are giving your body the right nourishment, at the right time.

This is part of what is called **Cycle Syncing**. Food is also a healthy and clever way of giving your body a natural remedy and relief from types of menstrual pain.

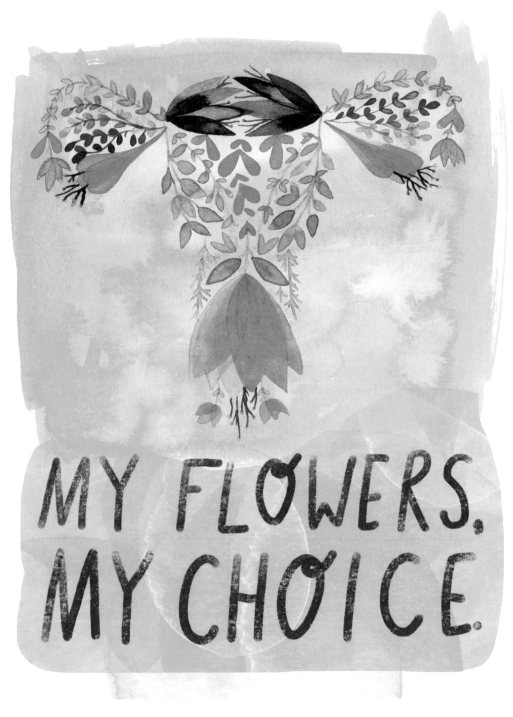

Artwork by Meera Lee Patel, "My Flowers My Choice", 2016

5

TRIAL PERIOD

When it comes to finding the right product, it's all about trial and error - and, above all, what works for YOU.

Nowadays there are so many products on the market that the supermarket aisle might be a bit overwhelming when it comes to knowing what to buy. Over the next few pages is a guide to the pros and cons of each product.

It's also worth reminding yourself that:

♦ You may want to use different products at different times of your period, depending on flow, and where you are going and what you're doing.

♦ What works for your sister/mum/auntie/best friend might not work for you. Remember, **all bodies are different** on the outside, as well as inside. Wearing a menstrual product should feel comfortable. If you're not, find a different one and ask your trusted adult for some help.

PADS
(absorb blood externally)

Types:
- Disposable or re-usable
- Variety of absorbency levels and sizes
- Back fastening with wings or clips, or without

Instructions:
Stick them onto the inside of your underwear. Fold wings back to stick underneath or clip buttons in place.

Why they're cool:
You see what's coming out of you. This way you can connect with your flow, blood colour and thickness, and keep an eye out for any changes

Not so cool for:
Swimming (they'll just absorb water)

Things to consider:
- For disposable: a cotton, non-scented, organic brand that doesn't contain plastic.

- For re-usable one that isn't white as it will look stained over time.

Disposal:
Disposable pads should be bagged and binned (never down the loo as they will block the pipes and may end up in the sea - eek!)

Re-usable pads should be rinsed with cold water and then air dried before being washed with the rest of your laundry.

Your health:
If you choose a disposable pad, consider using an organic cotton one as it will be free of bleach, scents and other chemicals, and healthier for your vulva.

The planet:
Re-usable pads won't create waste.

Approximate Cost:
Re-usable: £4-£6 per pad (or make your own! See page 140) **Disposable**: £3-£4 per pack of 10

TAMPONS
(absorb blood internally)

Types:
- Applicator tampons
- Non-applicator tampons

Instructions:
The applicator helps to insert the tampon into your vagina. Without, you will need to use a (clean) finger to push it in. You should not leave the applicator in your vagina - this should be disposed of in the bin, once used. The tampon cord should be left hanging out visibly so you can use it to gently pull out the tampon later. You should change a tampon every 4 hours.

Why they're cool:
Really useful for swimming and other types of exercise, as they absorb blood internally, so you won't feel blood coming out of you.

Not so cool for:
- A first time user. Inserting them can be a bit tricky initially, so it's all about experimenting.
- Seeing what's coming out of you.

Things to consider:
Choose the right size. If you pull it out and there are still sections of white visible, then you are using too large a size for your flow.

Disposal:
Bag it & bin it (no flushing!)

Your health:
Try to use an organic unbleached cotton tampon, as this is free from plastic and chemicals, and therefore healthier for your vagina.

The planet:
Consider a re-usable applicator. That way you are not disposing of unnecessary plastic or paper applicators after each use. They will need to be washed after use.

Approximate Cost:
75p - £3.50 a pack depending on quantity

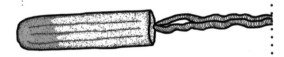

MENSTRUAL CUPS
(collect blood internally)

Types:
♦ Medical grade silicon or latex
♦ TPE-plastic *(not recommended)*

Sizing:
Menstrual cups vary in size depending on the brand you choose, so check the size guide on the packaging. Typically, there are 2 sizes: for those under 25, and for those over 25.

Why they're cool:
One cup is suitable for all flows. You can wear it hundreds of times and it will last up to 10 years. Winner!

   Obviously great for swimming and exercising as it's worn internally.

Not so cool for:
♦ A first-time user. Inserting them can be a bit tricky initially, so it's all about experimenting. Wear a panty liner too the first few times to check for leaks.

♦ Rinsing out in public loos or any cubicle that doesn't

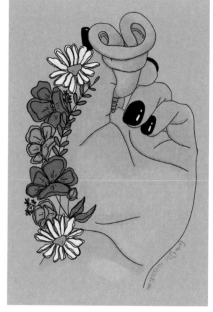

Artwork by Phiz, 'The 'C' fold', 2019

have a sink. You can get around this by bringing a bottle of water and rinsing it off over the loo.

Things to consider:
Buying a steriliser for your cup so that you can be sure it's properly cleaned every time.

Disposal:
None!

The planet:
There is zero waste as you are re-using it.

Approximate Cost:
£9-£25 depending on brands

HOW TO INSERT A MENSTRUAL CUP

WASH HANDS BEFORE AND AFTER

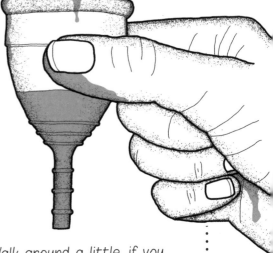

To insert:
This takes some practice! Make sure you have some privacy so you can take the time to experiment with inserting it correctly, without interruption.

- Practise folding your cup. There are several variations when it comes to folding. Look at the image below, can you guess which one is the 7 fold? The C fold? The 'push down' fold?

- Squat or lift one leg by placing it on the edge of your bath or toilet. Fold your cup and insert it into your vagina.

- Push it as high up as you can into your vagina, then slowly release the fold. You are trying to create suction so make sure the rim is round and sitting under your cervix. Adjust accordingly.

- Walk around a little, if you can feel it when you move, it's not suitably positioned, so try again.

Some cups are designed with a long stem that can be trimmed down for size. If you do so, just make sure you leave it long enough to be able to grab onto it.

To remove:
- Insert your finger to break the suction at the top of your vagina and then gently pull it out using the plug. **Do not drag the cup out** by pulling the plug only – you must break the suction for easy release.

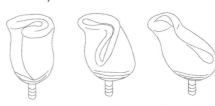

Artwork by Period Proof, 'The C, 7 and Push down Folds' 2019

RE-USABLE PANTS

(absorb blood externally)

Types:
Underwear, shorts, pants, leggings. All lined with ultra-thin micro-layers which are designed to absorb fluid

Instructions:
Just wear!

Why they're cool:
Super easy to use. They replace underwear and hold between 1-4 regular tampons worth of blood. Good for wearing at night.

Not so cool for:
Changing while you're out and about, although some pants are now being designed with poppers on the side for easy removal. Bring a wet bag if changed away from home.

Things to consider:
It takes some time to trust them! Initially it can feel odd to 'free bleed' into clothes...

Disposal:
None. They should be rinsed under a COLD tap until the water runs clear. Then air dry and put in a normal wash.

Your health:
Sorted

The planet:
Zero waste as you are re-using

Approximate Cost:
£10-£25

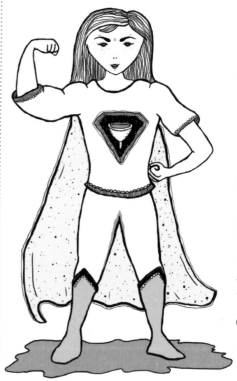

I can do bleeding.
What's your superhero power?

Thank you to Sarah Eichert for all her images in this section

THE BEST WAY TO MANAGE YOUR PERIOD

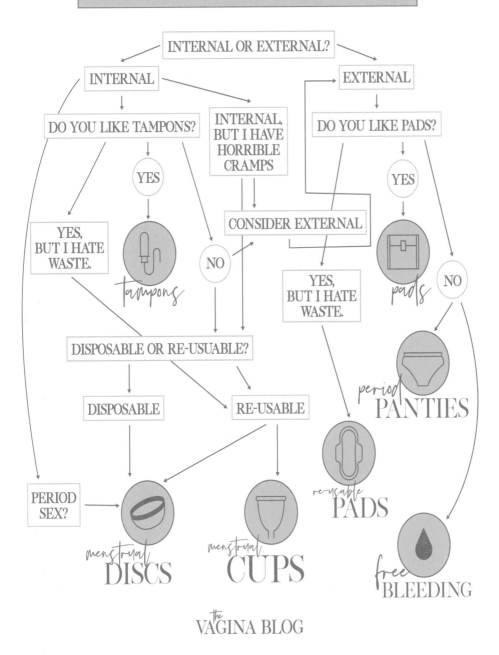

INTERNAL OR EXTERNAL?

INTERNAL

EXTERNAL

DO YOU LIKE TAMPONS?

INTERNAL, BUT I HAVE HORRIBLE CRAMPS

DO YOU LIKE PADS?

YES

YES

YES, BUT I HATE WASTE.

tampons

NO

CONSIDER EXTERNAL

pads

NO

YES, BUT I HATE WASTE.

DISPOSABLE OR RE-USUABLE?

period PANTIES

DISPOSABLE

RE-USABLE

PERIOD SEX?

re-usable PADS

menstrual DISCS

menstrual CUPS

free BLEEDING

the VAGINA BLOG

35

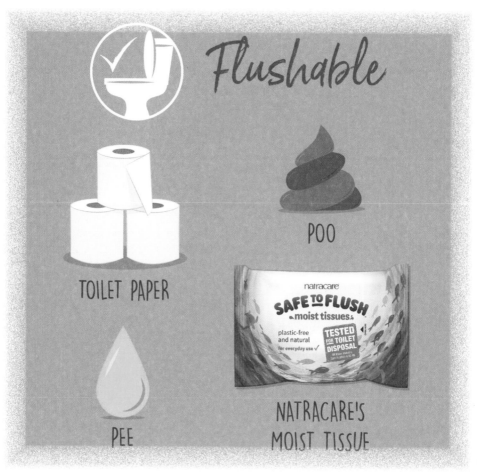

Artwork by Becky Reeves & Natracare

A Word on Disposal:

The image above makes it quite clear that, other than the 3P's (pee, poo and paper), absolutely nothing should be flushed down the loo. Natracare is the ONLY brand that have created biodegradable wet wipes which means they will disintegrate once watered down (confirmed by Anglia Water). Any other wet wipes won't break down and will create fatbergs (huge mountains of toilet waste that block sewers), causing the pipes to overflow and pollute our seas. This means huge problems for our beaches and ocean wildlife. So, the message is simple: **Bag it & Bin it!**

6

YOUR SUSTAINABLE PERIOD

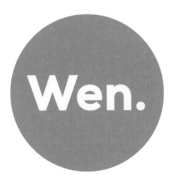

A word from the Women's Environmental Network:

The Problem: Menstrual taboos or period shaming has a massive impact on the products we use and how we dispose of them. Certain menstrual products can affect our health, end up in landfill, on our beaches, or pollute our oceans for decades. Could changing our attitude towards periods affect the choices we make about which menstrual products to use and how we dispose of them – which could then have a major impact on our health and environment?

Wen (Women's Environmental Network) has been campaigning on 'Environmenstrual' issues for over 30 years, providing information to girls, women and people who menstruate about the health and environmental impacts of menstrual products.

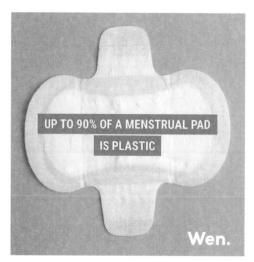

UP TO 90% OF A MENSTRUAL PAD IS PLASTIC

Wen.

Sustainable Products:

There are now disposable menstrual tampons and pads that do not contain plastic and are made from organic cotton. These disposable products work the same way as their mainstream counterparts that contain plastic. Natracare tampons and pads can even be composted in a home compost bin!

Menstrual cups cost between £10-£25 but last for around ten years - making them much more cost-effective in the long-term. There is also zero waste produced, apart from the materials used in the manufacturing process.

Re-usable pads work the same way as disposable pads. There are

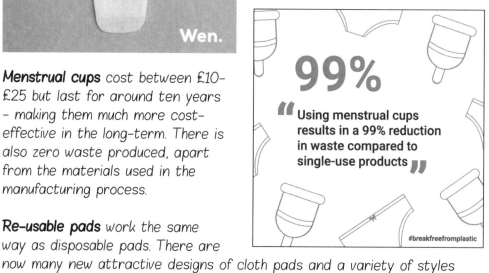

99%

" Using menstrual cups results in a 99% reduction in waste compared to single-use products "

#breakfreefromplastic

now many new attractive designs of cloth pads and a variety of styles and thickness to accommodate heavy and light periods. There are many new start-up businesses making cloth pads as this option is also gaining popularity, thanks to increased awareness around plastic pollution, waste and harmful chemicals in conventional disposable menstrual products.

Re-usable period pants are a relatively new addition to the reusable options. These are pants that can hold between two to four tampons' worth of blood. They are made from special material that absorbs the blood without making the pants too bulky. They are growing in popularity as people find them convenient and comfortable. They are especially popular for wearing at night, and for sports, if you are not comfortable with any of the internal options. They are relatively expensive, costing between £20-£30 per pair, but they last for many years.

ACTIVITY IDEA - Supermarket Sweep

Next time you're in your local supermarket, take a look at what menstrual products are available on the shelves. Are they mainly disposable? Or re-usable? What suggestions could you make, so that the supermarkets is able to improve the selection of products available to customers?

ACTIVITY IDEA - Menstrual expenses!

Ask a family member or friend who menstruates what menstrual product they have used since starting their period. How much does that product cost? Work out what they have spent on periods in their whole lives. Yikes! What savings could YOU make?

THE HORMONAL ROLLERCOASTER

FEELING ON TOP OF THE WORLD!

GIVE ME ALL THE CHOCOLATE

SPOTS GALORE

FEELING HORNY

SNAPPED AT A FRIEND

HIT A LOW POINT

It's a bloody ride!

Artwork by Hazel Mead, 'The Hormonal Rollercoaster', 2019

7

A DIFFICULT
PERIOD

All the changes that your body is going through in the run-up to or during your monthly bleed may cause you some discomfort. This is known as Pre Menstrual Syndrome or P.M.S.

Essentially the discomfort is caused by **hormonal changes** that may trigger symptoms that will include cramps, bloating and fatigue, tender breasts and acne. It's also common to feel low and sensitive during your winter phase. Take it easy on yourself and really try tuning into what your body feels able to cope with and what your body is telling you at this time of the month.

All of these significant changes happening inside and outside of your body are activated by hormones. The best way of describing them is as substances that send messages to your body to make changes. They are also responsible for any changes in feelings and emotions. Now you know who to blame!

Just as human beings have different hair, eyes and body shapes, **people react differently to hormones**. So, while your best friend always seems to feel GREAT (frustratingly for you) and has no skin conditions, you might be really suffering with fluctuations in mood, but also displaying physical signs of puberty that you are struggling to manage.

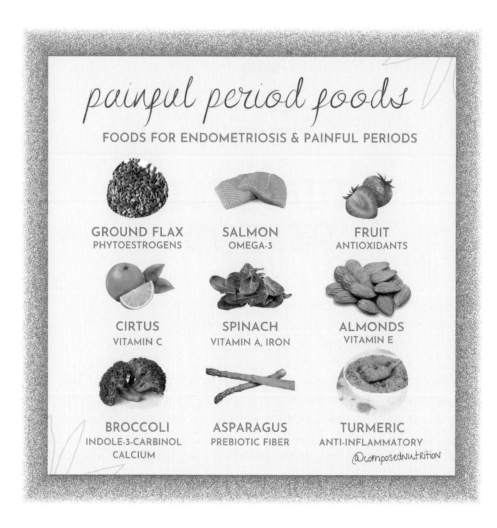

painful period foods

FOODS FOR ENDOMETRIOSIS & PAINFUL PERIODS

GROUND FLAX
PHYTOESTROGENS

SALMON
OMEGA-3

FRUIT
ANTIOXIDANTS

CIRTUS
VITAMIN C

SPINACH
VITAMIN A, IRON

ALMONDS
VITAMIN E

BROCCOLI
INDOLE-3-CARBINOL
CALCIUM

ASPARAGUS
PREBIOTIC FIBER

TURMERIC
ANTI-INFLAMMATORY

@composednutrition

Artwork by Krista King, 'Painful Periods', 2020

Take action:

Go back to your list of trusted adults. They'll have been through this, just like you! If you are experiencing strong physical symptoms (such as terrible acne, or a sudden increase in body odour) tell them, as there are easy one-step solutions.

It may feel awkward at first, but it will be a huge relief! If talking is too difficult, consider writing it down and leaving it somewhere for them to find.

Artwork by Vanessa, 'When you feel sad...', 2019

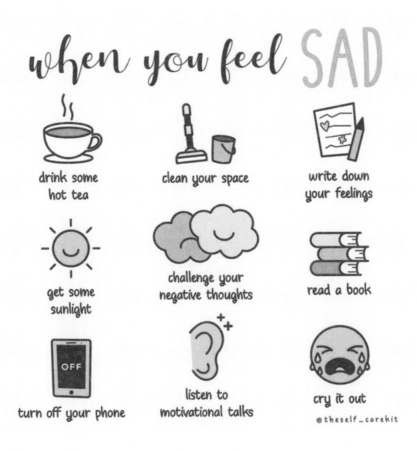

when you feel SAD

drink some hot tea

clean your space

write down your feelings

get some sunlight

challenge your negative thoughts

read a book

turn off your phone

listen to motivational talks

cry it out

@theself_carekit

P.M.S. can vary from person to person. If you're finding your symptoms difficult to manage, do speak to your trusted adult about this as you might need some support - especially if you have a challenging day ahead, or pressures at school to deal with. There are some things you can do to make yourself feel a little better.

Give these yoga positions illustrated overleaf a try, as they will get the blood moving gently, whilst also making sure it's headed south.

43

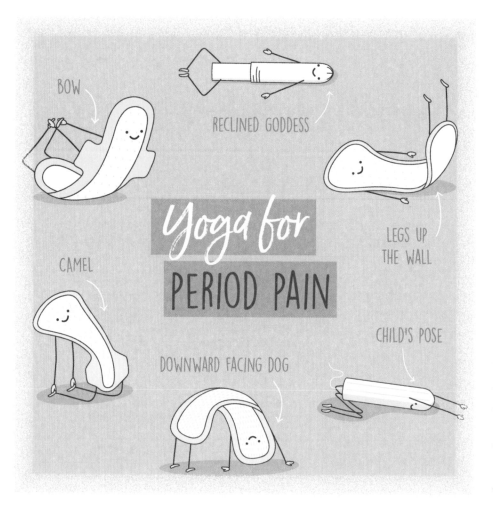

BOW

RECLINED GODDESS

Yoga for

PERIOD PAIN

CAMEL

LEGS UP THE WALL

CHILD'S POSE

DOWNWARD FACING DOG

Artwork by Becky Greeves at Natracare, 2019

P.M.S. Self-Care Hints and Tips

Clothing: Loose, comfortable clothing that will make you feel snug and cosy. If you're wearing a bra, taking it off will make you feel freer. If you're cold, keep your feet warm.

Oils: Lavender, clove, ylang-ylang, rose and peppermint are recommended for P.M.S. A few drops can be massaged into the abdominal area, or infused into the room through a diffuser, or simply rubbed onto palms and temples for a soothing smell.

Drink: WATER! You can't drink enough.

Food: see the chart on the previous page.

Recommended extras: Hot water bottle (warm, not boiling hot), creature comforts (if you have a pet, snuggle up), sofa + Netflix.

If you can indulge…go for it.

And let's not forget…SLEEEEEEEP!

What symptoms have you experienced? Write them down here:

Physical ....

....

....

....

Emotional ....

....

....

....

Remedies that have worked for you:

....

....

....

....

When to see your doctor

If in doubt about any aspect of your menstrual cycle, please speak to your trusted adult, or speak directly to your doctor. It goes without saying that there is no such thing as a silly question when it comes to our bodies. Your health matters more than anything!

Below are just a few of the reasons why it might be a good idea to make an appointment:

- Bleeding outside of your menstruation phase. If you experience any kind of unusual bleeding during your cycle, it is worth having this checked out.

- If you haven't had a period for more than 90 days.

- If you experience very heavy bleeding.

- If you have 'funny' smelling discharge as this may be a possible sign of infection.

- You have a niggling feeling that something's up. You know your body, so get the peace of mind and make an appointment

A word on Pain

It is entirely normal for menstruation to be uncomfortable due to cramping. However, if you are in agony month after month, and taking large amounts of pain relief, this could be a sign that you are suffering with a condition that needs attention. Make an appointment for your peace of mind.

How to get comfortable before and during a medical appointment

- Ask a friend or trusted adult to come along with you. It can be a little awkward talking to a stranger about a very personal aspect of our life, as well as being overwhelming taking all the information in. Bringing someone along to be your 'ears' is hugely helpful and supportive.

- Ask for a female practitioner.

- Practise what you are going to say, or even better, write it down.

- Make notes during the appointment.

- Remember that there is a confidentiality agreement between you and your doctor, so you can be open and honest. Get to know your doctor so that you can begin to build a relationship with him/her.

EXERCISING ON YOUR PERIOD
MAY SEEM A LITTLE BLEAK
WITH POSSIBLE BRA NIPPLE CHAFING
AND THE RISK OF A LEAK
HOWEVER GIVE IT A GO
IF YOU'RE FEELING A LITTLE BLUE
AS IT'S GREAT FOR PESKY CRAMPS
AND WILL BOOST YOUR MOOD TOO!

Poetic periods Artwork by Holly Lehmann, 'Exercising', 2019

8

P.E. PERIOD

There are no hard and fast rules, and you can pretty much do anything you like while you menstruate. It really just depends on how you feel and how your body feels. If you feel like going trampolining, do it. If, however, you are feeling very fragile, then it is more than acceptable to excuse yourself from P.E.

If you are committed to doing P.E. at school or you have a swimming gala that you just can't get out of, here are some tips to make it as comfortable as possible:

- If you are running, swimming or doing any physical activity that requires you to wear tight clothing such as gymnastics, you might want to consider an internal product such as a tampon or menstrual cup.

- If you're running long distances and don't want to use an internal product, period pants will feel more comfortable than pads as they act as underwear, rather than an additional layer, and will prevent any kind of rash caused by rubbing.

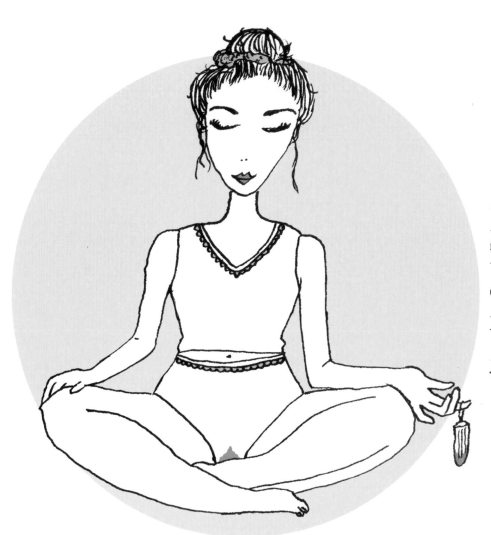

Artwork by Sarah Eichart

⚬ Talk to your trusted adult about pain relief if you are experiencing a heavy flow and need to exert yourself physically.

⚬ Tell the person in charge. Find a trusted teacher who you can talk to and just let them know that you are menstruating. This way they will know to expect a bit less of you today (as well as be impressed with your honesty and perseverance!).

⚬ If you're practising Yoga, it might be worth avoiding inverse positions (where you are upside down), or staying in them for too long. This is because while you are menstruating your blood flow is following gravity and heading out of your system, and inverting may restrict or disrupt the direction of flow.

Some inspiring facts around athletes and menstruation

26 year-old Kiran Ghandi made the decision to 'free bleed' her way through 26.2 miles when running the London Marathon. By the time she realised she was going to be menstruating, she didn't see how she was going to be able to change her tampon, so she thought 'why not?' No shame!

Chelsea Women were the first football club in the world to tailor their training programme around players' menstrual cycles in an attempt to enhance performance and cut down on injuries.

Japanese swimmer Fu Yuanhui hit the headlines when she lost the 4 x 100 metres relay in 2016 at the Rio Olympics swimming race and publicly blamed her loss on the fact that she was on her period. She went on to win the Bronze medal for the 100m backstroke. Whoop!

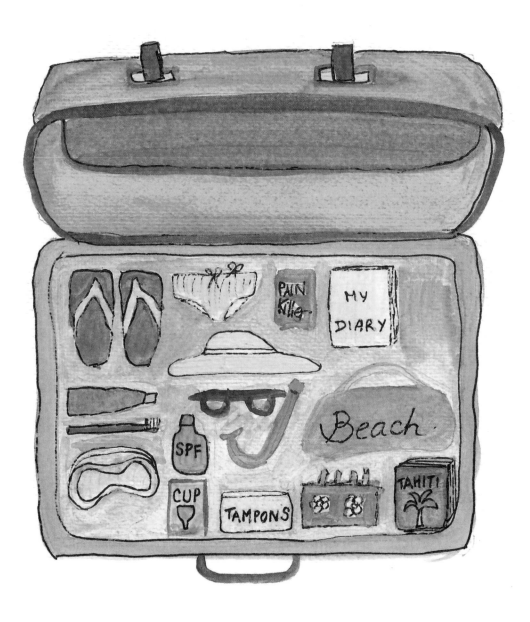

9

HOLIDAY
PERIOD

The holiday is booked! Hooray! Then it dawns on you there is a chance you might start menstruating whilst you are supposed to be diving into the sea and hanging out by the pool with your friends....

Don't worry, there are a few options that are worth considering:

1. Use an internal menstrual product. It is worth playing around with what you feel comfortable with before leaving for the beach, as inserting it correctly requires some experimenting. See the table on page 35 about tampons and menstrual cups to see which option suits you better.

2. Use period-proof swimwear. This works the same way as period-proof underwear as it absorbs blood. It's new to the market so you might want to test it out in the bath first!

DONT FORGET! *Take your remedies for period pain with you on holiday as it might be hard to find exactly what you need abroad.*

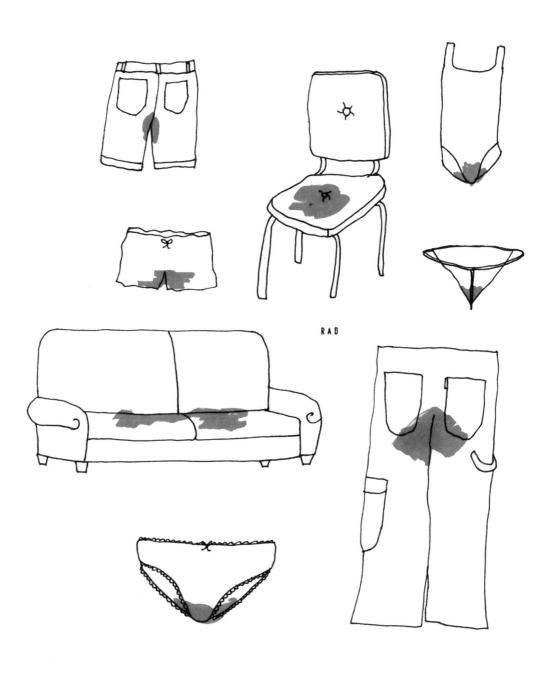

Artwork by Rachel Duggan, 2019

10

PERIOD PIECE

Bloody Leaks

There is not a person in the world who menstruates, who hasn't bled through clothes, onto chairs, freshly pressed white sheets, carseats, cushions, sofas... You name it, it's happened. Naturally this can feel SO embarrassing. If this happens in a public place, try to find a trusted adult who can help you, while you sort yourself out. And then follow our instructions on the next page on how to remove blood stains.

Just remember that you won't be the first, nor the last!

Don't panic. Find a coat, jumper or item of clothing to wrap around your waist and excuse yourself. If you've leaked onto the seat, then cover the stain temporarily with a paper or bag to deal with later.

Once in a toilet if you can't get hold of a menstrual product, roll up some tissue and place it in your underwear. It will buy you some time until you find something.

Bloody stains

What you need:
- *Blood-stained item of clothing*
- <u>**Cold**</u> *water tap*
- *Somewhere to hang item to dry*

<u>Instructions:</u>
- Let the cold tap run on the stain for as long as possible. If it doesn't come off, leave it to soak in cold water.
Hot water will set the blood into the fabric. Only use cold.

- Once stain-free, wring it out and leave it to dry. If you're not at home, place the item in a bag to take home.

- If the stain persists, you'll need something stronger and for that you'll need your trusted adult or trusted supermarket to find a stain remover.

- If the stain is on a sofa cushion or fabric and you are somewhere public then you can attempt to scrub or soak, but it's worth coming clean (!) and 'fessing up' to a friendly-looking adult for help, or to anyone who looks like they might menstruate (because they will be experienced in this field!).

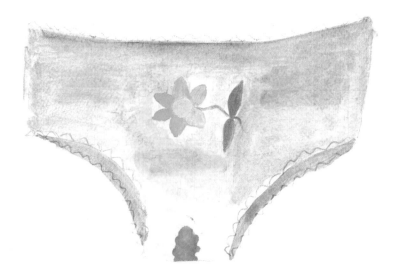

Artwork By Kat Cass, 'Period Euphemisms', 2019

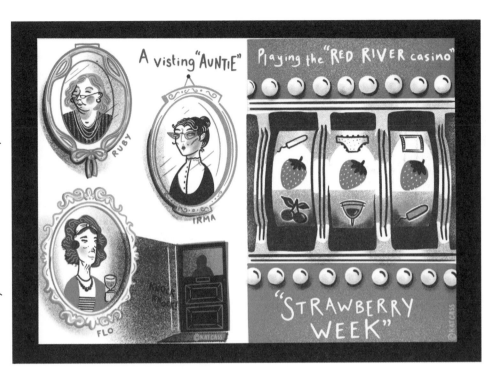

Period Euphemisms

Auntie Flo. Rag Week. Shark Week. Being On. Moontime. Aunty Flow. Mother Nature. Having The Painters In. Leak Week. Blood Rain. The Bleedies. Seeing Red. Ladies Day. Joined The Red Cross. Japanese Flag Week. Little Red Friend. Bloody Mary. Time Of The Month. Monthlies. Code Red. Strawberry Fields. Kitty's Got A Nose-bleed. Luna Phase. The Big Red Bus. Painters Are In. Arsenal Are Playing At Home. Red Sea. On the Blob. Riding The Cotton Unicorn. Riding the Crimson Wave...

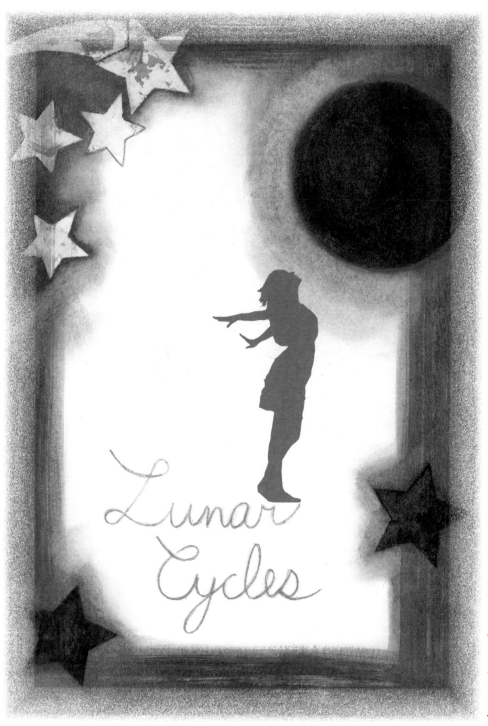

Artwork by Sara J Beazley, 'Lunar Cycles', 2019

11

SUPER-POWER PERIOD

You will have noticed that most of the code words for period on the previous page are not always positive. In order to understand why there is such 'bad blood' associated with menstruation, we need to take a trip in our time machine...

In Ancient times, when the moon was the only source of light after sunset, it is believed that women would gather under the light of a new moon to celebrate their monthly bleed. This was because their menstrual cycles were in sync with the cycles of the moon, known as lunar cycles. (In fact the term 'menstruation' comes from the Greek word 'mene', which means moon).

Just as the moon takes 28 days to circle the Earth, a woman's cycle is approximately the same. They believed that their periods were what connected them to nature, to Earth and to the seasons. This connection between women and the moon was seen as sacred, and women tapped into what each phase brought to their lives.

The time of the month when women bled was seen as a very empowering time. Their link to the moon and the energy they created as gathered women was so strong - perhaps so much so, that it is believed men saw this superpower as something to be scared and wary of! And this was the beginning of the scaremongering story around periods...

With the rise of technology and, more importantly artificial light, the connection between women and the lunar cycles has been interrupted. However, some women will still claim to be in sync with the moon and it is not uncommon to find that women who live together or in close proximity are in sync with each other. So, the connection remains, on some level.

For centuries women in society have had to hide the fact that they are bleeding, and this secrecy has caused longstanding stigma and taboo. Sadly, there are still some countries today where a huge amount of fear around periods remains. In some parts of India for instance, girls and women are sent to 'Menstrual Huts' for the length of their monthly bleed as they are considered to be dirty and unhygienic. Some girls even see themselves as cursed.

It's time to reclaim the superpower that was celebrated centuries ago. Some women see their menstrual cycle as an internal compass or a clock, and perceive it as a window to view their inner world. The new moon in their lives (the bleeding part of the cycle) is also an opportunity to start over and refresh. It's a new cycle, a new phase, a new beginning!

Below are some more positive ways to describe the fact that you are bleeding. Feel free to add or make up your own!

ACTIVITY IDEA- Positive Euphemisms

Can you think of some positive code words to describe the fact that you are bleeding? Feel free to make up your own!

Here are some suggestions:

I'm on my period. Period.

. . . .

I'm going with the flow.

. . . .

It's winter.

. . . .

It's moontime.

12

PERIOD DRAMA

There are SO many myths and misconceptions around menstruation! So, let's address this unnecessary drama. Here are just a few that oh-so-desperately need busting.

- Periods are dirty
- If you swim whilst on your period you will be eaten by a shark
- You shouldn't cook or touch food whilst menstruating
- If you use an internal menstrual product (eg. tampon or menstrual cup), you are no longer a virgin
- People can tell when you are on your period
- You can hold in your period
- If you wee, you need to take your tampon out
- Irregular periods are a bad sign
- PMS is not real – it's all in our heads
- You need to wash your vagina with products

ALL ABSOLUTE RUBBISH!

Periods are dirty
Periods are a natural part of our biological make-up. In fact, they are a great sign that your body is developing as it should. If one considers this scientifically, in order for an embryo to implant and develop, it would

need to do so in an environment that's free from any toxins. So, in actual fact, menstrual blood is as clean as it gets. Anyone who believes that periods are dirty should hear that their existence alone relies on someone menstruating at some point. At this point, just over 200 million people worldwide are on their period. They can't all possibly be dirty.

If you swim whilst on your period you will be eaten by a shark
It is absolutely fine and safe to go swimming whilst bleeding. It may be preferable to use a tampon or cup - for your comfort, but not because of sharks! Sharks will not detect if are bleeding in the ocean so swim free… and it may even relieve your cramps.

You shouldn't cook or touch food whilst menstruating
Sadly, this myth is deeply embedded in some cultures where periods are seen as dirty and unhygienic. Although some countries are still suffering with stigmas around periods, as well as period poverty, there is a huge effort being made by charities and campaigners to try and change this to a more positive narrative. Needless to say, this myth is absolutely untrue: there is nothing you can't do whilst bleeding, including cooking (and touching plants is also fine fyi).

If you use an internal menstrual product (eg. tampon or menstrual cup) you are no longer a virgin
This depends on how you define 'virginity'. Most people consider themselves to be a virgin until the first time they have penetrative sex, which tends to be associated with the tearing of the hymen, a thin tissue that's located inside your vagina. But the truth is that there is a much wider view of what sex is these days (not just penis in vagina sex), and also everyone's hymen is different. Generally speaking, the hymen will stretch and eventually break when it needs to, and it's very unlikely this is due to a tampon or cup.

People can tell when you are on your period
Nope. What sometimes occurs is that people may suspect you are bleeding for a variety of reasons that are annoying: if you are in a bad mood, sluggish, grumpy, etc…but that is nothing more than a GUESS. There is definitely no way of people knowing, by looking at you, that you are menstruating. We also want to add to this one: and if they do, SO WHAT?!

You can hold in your period

There is no stopping menstrual blood. Unlike urine, which comes out of your urethra which has sphincter muscles (like elastic bands), menstrual blood comes out of your vagina where there is no sphincter muscle. Your vagina is an open tunnel headed south. It may certainly look like you are peeing blood when you go to the loo, as only a small amount of blood changes the colour of urine. Also. Don't hold in wee for longer than you need to.

If you need a wee you need to take your tampon out

You do not need to take out your tampon when you urinate. As discussed above urine and blood exit through different holes. (See page 9 for a reminder of the function of the different holes in the vulva).

PMS is not real, it's all in our heads

Haha. Not funny. The lining of our uterus sheds entirely over the course of a week, accompanied by a huge change in hormones, and we're not allowed to feel anything? (exhale deeply…). Justifying it here would just feed into the myth, so silence is golden. And PMS is real.

On a serious note, if you are suffering with any sort of pain, talk to your trusted adult. It's possible the solution is simple, such as an over-the-counter remedy at the chemist. If the situation persists, talk to your doctor.

Irregular periods are a bad sign

When you are just starting your period, it is normal for it to take years to regulate. For instance, if you start your first period when you are 14, it is natural for it to be irregular for at least 2 years. Once your cycle is established and regular however, there are many reasons for irregular periods - such as weight change, travelling long haul, diet, stress and, of course, pregnancy. Also try to keep in mind that if you are going through a difficult time at home or sitting exams for instance, the timing and flow of your period may be affected.

You need to wash your vagina with products

Your vulva and vagina are self-cleaning! It is not necessary for you to wash out, clean, steam, douche or shower inside the vulva. The body has an amazing way of cleansing itself. All that is required is that you keep the outside clean by giving the outer lips of the vulva and anal area a general wash, rinse and dry. Whilst you are on your period, just wash the outside of the vulva, but not inside. Your body has a magical way of getting rid of every last drop of blood. So why all the products at the chemist to clean 'private parts'? Ah! Good question. Many useless products exist (another book).

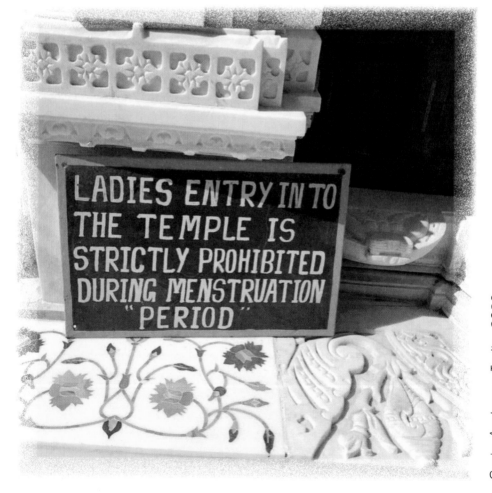

Susie Anglesey, India, 2020

13

PERIODS AROUND THE WORLD

Some cultures have incredible resources for coping with their monthly bleed:

- In Uganda, goat skin is used to absorb blood. Women wrap the material around their waist and position it between their legs a bit like a nappy. This tradition has been passed down through generations. It is also common to 'simply' sit over a hole in the ground so that the blood falls into it.
- Nyanda, a small piece of cloth used as a menstrual pad in Malawi, is placed inside underwear to absorb blood. Rinsing can be problematic if there is no free-flowing water.
- In Zambia they collect cotton from the fields, roll it up and place it in their underwear.
- In Nepal, women are increasingly making their own re-usable menstrual pads using traditional Nepalese fabrics.
- In India cow patties (yes, cow poo) are moulded into shape, wrapped in a rag and used as pads.
- In Mali, Africa, women spend their periods in menstrual huts as people believe they are not clean whilst they are bleeding. Some charities such as Amnesty International are working towards banning such practices.

The picutre on the left shows one of many temples in India that prohibit people who are menstruating from entering their place of worship.

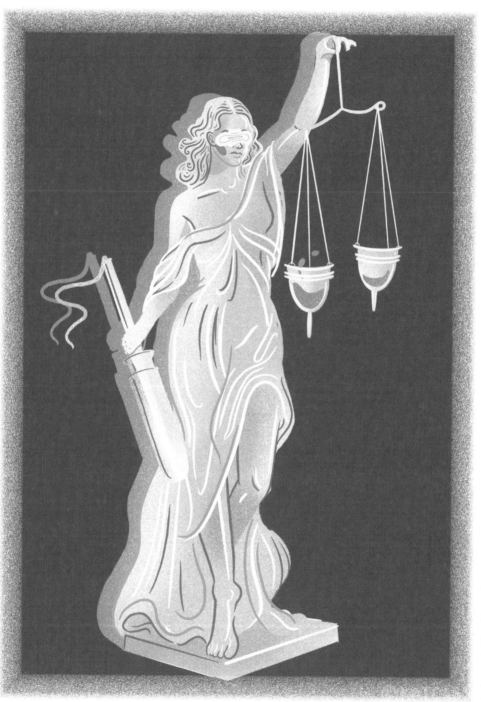

Artwork By Kat Cass, 'Lady Justice', 2019

14

PERIOD POVERTY

Period Poverty refers to not being able to access menstrual products for financial reasons.

Plan UK, a children's rights charity, have this to say: "If we're to put an end to period poverty here in the UK then we need to tackle the 'toxic trio' of issues at the root of the problem – namely the high cost of period products, the stigma and shame surrounding periods, and a lack of education about what makes a healthy period." In 2019, Plan Uk found that:

- Nearly half (48%) of girls aged 14-21 in the UK are embarrassed by their periods
- 1 in 7 (14%) girls admit they did not know what was happening when they started their period, and more than a quarter (26%) report that they did not know what to do when it happened
- Only 1 in 5 (20%) girls feel comfortable discussing their period with their teacher
- Almost three quarters (71%) of girls admit that they have felt embarrassed buying menstrual products
- 40% of girls have had to use toilet roll because they can't afford proper menstrual products
- Almost 70% of girls in the UK aren't allowed to go to the toilet during school lesson time

Thankfully the tide is changing. We can, as the movement to 'free periods' grows stronger, begin to talk more openly about menstruation, after hundreds of years of keeping it under wraps. Phew.

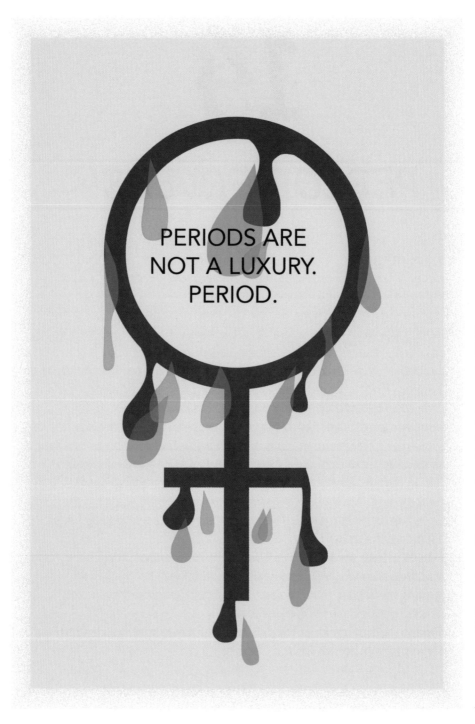

PERIODS ARE
NOT A LUXURY.
PERIOD.

Artwork by Dhillon Kaur, 'Periods Are Not A Luxury', 2019

15

FREE PERIODS

At this point in time, there are some positive changes that are worth feeling good about, that are freeing up the conversation around menstruation. Good news!

- Thanks to Plan International UK we now have a Period Emoji. Now you can tell all your friends that you're on your period with the touch of a button!
- 'Tampon Tax' has been abolished. Thanks to a fantastic campaign initiated by Laura Coryton, the Government has pledged to lift the tax on all menstrual products (not just tampons, as the tax is called, but all products) as they are no longer regarded as a luxury, but rather a life essential.
- The Government has also pledged to provide menstrual products to all schools to tackle period poverty, ensuring everyone has access to them. This was led by 'Free Periods' campaigner Amika George.
- Supermarkets are being urged to offer a wider range of healthier and more sustainable products on their shelves thanks to period campaigner Ella Daish.
- Way to go New York! Officially the first state in the U.S.A. to require period product makers to disclose ingredients. There are calls for UK manufacturers to do the same. We have a right to know what we are placing under or in our vaginas. That way, we can all have healthier, happier and more environmentally friendly periods.

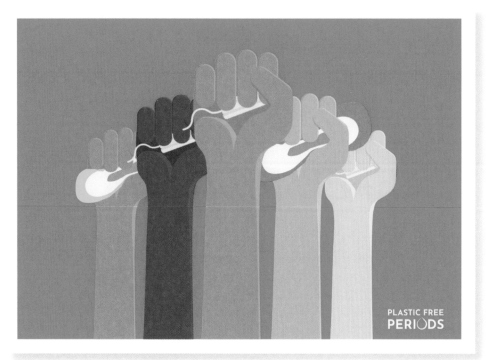

Artwork by City to Sea, 'Plastic Free Periods', 2019

TAKE ACTION

Talk about MENSTRUAL not SANITARY products. *('Sanitary' implies there is something unhygienic about bleeding once a month.)*

Talk to your form teacher or your PSHE teacher about period education. *City to Sea are at present offering free period training for teachers. Ask your teacher to enquire about the Rethink Periods training programme.*

<u>**If you feel brave enough...**</u>
Be honest about how you feel. *Name it! It might help you to be open, as well as inspire those around you to share emotions around menstruation. If you are frustrated, sad or angry, your 'blood sisters' will share your pain with compassion and understanding.*

Tackle taboos and address misconceptions. Don't be afraid to calmly challenge anyone who you feel is demonising periods. Remember that periods are entirely normal, natural and healthy, and there is nothing to be ashamed of, particularly if millions of people on Earth menstruating at this very moment!

ACTIVITY IDEAS -
Period education at school

Talk to your form teacher or school nurse about doing some of the following:

1. Designing a period mascot

2. Writing a song/rap/poem

3. If you think products could be better distributed, make a suggestion to the person in charge and create signposts around the school.

GLUE

4. Designing a poster for the school toilets as a reminder to only flush the 3Ps

Some ideas for slogans and tag lines:

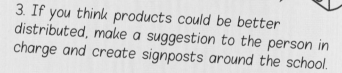

Go With The Flow   Bloody Break   Free Periods!

Blood Sisters   Period Power   No Bad Blood

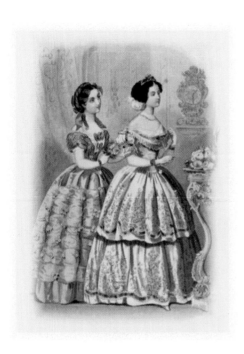

16

PERIODS IN HISTORY

And soon after that, the first disposable pad was introduced.

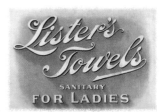

1800's • **1890** • • • • • • • • • • • • • • **1929** • • • • • •

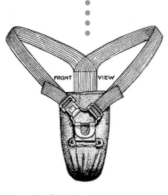

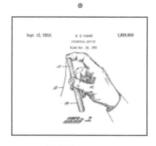

In the **1800s**, 'free bleeding' was quite common. Women would just bleed through their clothes. It was thought they would sometimes wear the same clothes from the start of their period, to the end. Eeek!

In **1890** Hoosier's Sanitary Belt (above) was developed - a belt to which women could pin washable cloth pads.

In **1929** Dr Earle Haas created the first tampon (above) after getting the idea from a woman who was inserting a sponge into her vagina to absorb the blood.

It's interesting to take a look back throughout history to see how women coped in the past with their monthly bleed. One thing is clear, they were very resourceful! We sadly don't have that much information about this time, as most of it was recorded by men! HIStory... hmmm.

In **1937**, Leona Chalmers invented the first menstrual cup (right) made from latex rubber. She was the first woman to invent something in this field, following a long line of men who had previously done so. Bravo!

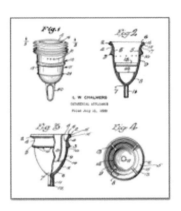

1937 .... **1957** .... **1970s** ..... **Now**

In **1957**, Mary Kenner, a self-taught inventor, invented the first ever patent for a belt to secure sanitary napkins

This was a huge step for women in terms of preventing leaks and stains.

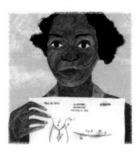

Self-adhesive pads came onto the market

Healthier and greener products to choose from!

<u>More fascinating menstrual facts</u>:

- Ancient Egyptians soaked papyrus in the River Nile and then made tampons out of the sheets. They also drank red wine to ritualise the connection with menstrual blood and spiritual power. Cheers!

- Ancient Greeks used menstrual blood to fertilise crops to symbolise growth during springtime festivals. They also made tampons from bits of wood with lint wrapped around them.

- In Medieval Times, women used to burn toads and keep the ashes in a little pouch on their stomachs as they believed it relieved them of aches and pains. They used rags as pads.

- The Romans used wool to soak up the blood.

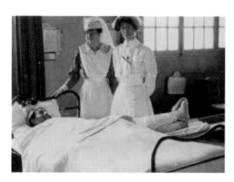

- During the First World War, French nurses borrowed bandages from wounded soldiers to make their own menstrual pads - and that was the beginning of the first pads available on the market by Kotex.

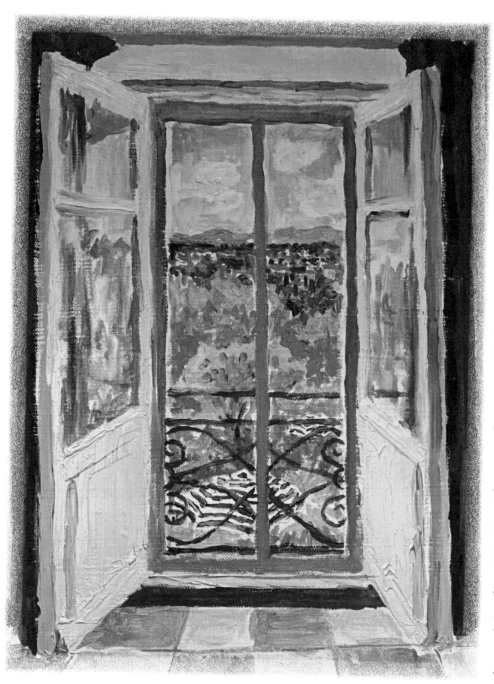

Artwork by Alex Uxbridge, 'A view in Provence' 2018

You can learn a lot about yourself from your period...

Section 2

Tuning in to your cycle

· ·

Name: ....

Age: .... Date of birth: ....

I got my first period on: ....

· ·

This is what happened when I first got my period: (Where were you? Who were you with and what happened?) ....

....

....

....

....

....

THIS PERIOD IN MY LIFE

Trusted adults I can talk to about periods:

- ....
- ....
- ....

People around me who menstruate:

- ....
- ....
- ....

What I know about periods:
(It's ok if you don't know much, that's why you have this book!)

....

....

....

....

....

....

....

....

....

....

....

HOW TO USE THIS SECTION

In this section you will have the opportunity to tune into YOUR menstrual cycle: its flow and your feelings.

In the previous section you will have learnt about all the super-powers in each phase of your cycle. This section gives you the opportunity to apply the information to your own life, making the most of each phase and seeing what it brings.

<u>What's the point in tracking your cycle?</u>
As well as the obvious reason of just getting to know your body and yourself better, tracking your period is useful for other reasons:

1. It's one of the few external signs we have to gauge our own fertility and our health generally, and can be seen as a sign that your body is in working order.

2. Linking your phases to seasons is a great way of seeing how you evolve across the course of a menstrual cycle, and to connect deeper with what your body is going through.

3. Medically, you well may be asked by a doctor if your periods are regular, and to describe the flow, pain, or amount of blood lost. There is no expectation to have to remember it all, so tracking is useful for that reason.

4. Knowing what season (phase) you're in makes communication easier with loved ones. If you say you are in Winter, perhaps they'll know to treat you a little more gently at this time!

You're all set! Take a look at these useful tools on the following pages:
- A feelings wheel
- A menstrual blood colour chart
- An annual lunar chart
- Plenty of monthly flow charts for you to complete
- 2 Periods of the Year tables

The Feelings Wheel

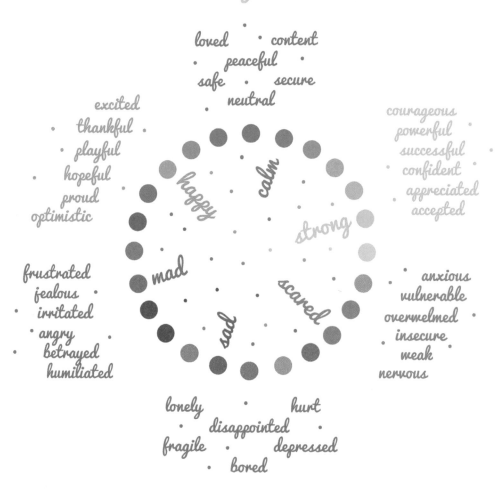

loved · content
peaceful ·
safe · secure
neutral

excited
thankful
playful
hopeful
proud
optimistic

courageous
powerful
successful
confident
appreciated
accepted

happy

calm

strong

mad

scared

sad

anxious
vulnerable
overwelmed
insecure
weak
nervous

frustrated
jealous
irritated
angry
betrayed
humiliated

lonely · hurt
disappointed
fragile · depressed
bored

Artwork by Carotte et Compagnie, 'The Feelings Wheel' 2020

THE FEELINGS WHEEL

Your period brings about so many changes in the way we feel and sometimes it can be very difficult to try to find the right words to describe them. This wheel has been colour-coded so that each emotion is linked to a colour, and then broken down into a more detailed description.

Feelings are linked to your psychological and emotional state, which is separate from the physical pain that you experience in your body. This wheel allows you to separate the two, focusing on emotional wellbeing.

True Colours

If you can't decide on a single word to put into your chart, feel free to fill in the space in the colour that best represents your feelings. Once you have completed an entire monthly chart in colour, it can be useful to look back and observe any colour patterns or recurring emotions throughout the month.

what does the colour of your period mean?

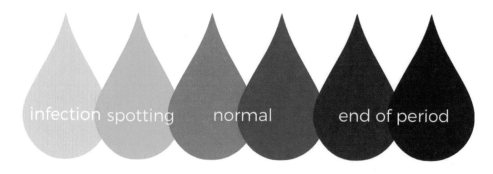

infection spotting normal end of period

are clots normal?
clots are chunky, jelly like red blobs
small, occasional clots = normal
large, frequent clots = abnormal

how much blood is lost during menstruation?
average flow is 30-50 ml
heavy flow is over 80 ml

Artwork by Crystal Kennings 'What does the colour of your period mean?', 2019

MENSTRUAL BLOOD COLOUR CHART

During your menstruation phase, it is normal for blood to vary in colour throughout the 3-7 days that you bleed. Opposite is a menstrual blood colour chart.

Colour: Opposite is a guide only. If you experience any other symptoms such as an odd smell, unusually heavy bleeding, or more pain than usual, make sure you tell your trusted adult or see your doctor, as it may be a sign of an infection.

Smell: It is entirely normal for period blood to smell. If you are using a pad or pants you will inevitably be exposed to the smell of period blood. If, however, the smell changes or seems unusually fishy or strong, tell your trusted adult or see your doctor.

Oh, and poo: In the run-up to and during your period, you may have looser stools, or experience some constipation. This is entirely normal and is due to hormonal changes. Drinking lots of water is the best thing you can do to help move your stools along comfortably and to stay hydrated.

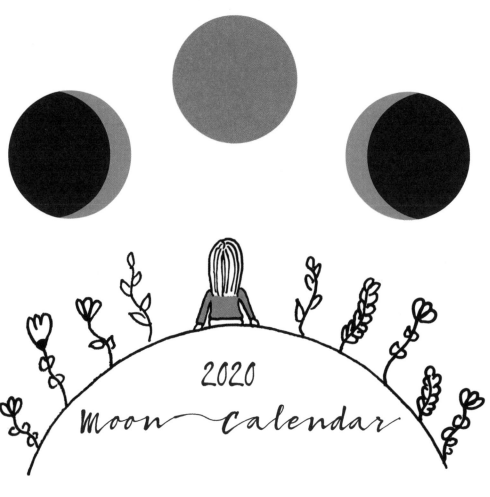

2020

Moon Calendar

ʒaɴ	2 ◐	10 ○	17 ◑	24 ●		ʒuʟ	4 ○	12 ◐	20 ●	27 ◑	
ꜰᴇʙ	1 ◐	8 ○	15 ◑	23 ●		auɢ	3 ○	11 ◐	18 ●	25 ◑	
maʀ	2 ◐	9 ○	16 ◑	24 ●		sᴇʀ	1 ○	10 ◐	17 ●	23 ◑	
aʀʀ	1 ◐	7 ○	14 ◑	22 ●	30 ◐	ocт	1 ○	9 ◐	16 ●	23 ◑	31 ○
may	7 ○	14 ◐	22 ●	29 ◑		nov	8 ◐	14 ●	21 ◑	30 ○	
ʒuɴ	5 ○	13 ◐	20 ●	28 ◑		ᴅᴇc	7 ◐	14 ●	21 ◑	29 ○	

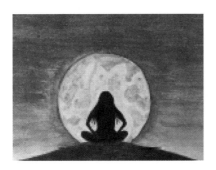

ANNUAL LUNAR CHART

In the monthly charts there is space around the outside to plot the phase of the moon. Please read the chapter on Super Power Period in Section 1 to remind yourself of the history around menstruation and its synchronisation with the cycles of the moon.

On the opposite page is an annual lunar chart for you to locate the exact date of the phases of the moon throughout the year. This information is useful so that you may observe and keep track of any potential synchronisation with your own cycle and the moon! Imagine being able to look at the moon and work out when your next period is due! Super power or what?

THE CHART HERE IS FOR 2020 ONLY. WE HAVE INLCUDED A 2021 CHART IN THE 'BONUS MATERIAL' SECTION ON PAGE 138 AND OTHERS CAN EASILY BE FOUND ONLINE

MONTHLY CHART

Here is an example of a completed monthly chart:

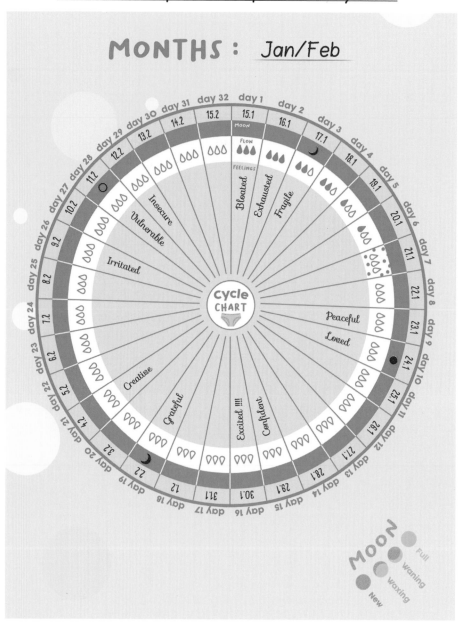

On the following pages are two years worth of monthly charts. Each chart represents one menstrual cycle, typically lasting for between 27 and 32 days. The circle allows you to plot all the information relating to your period, and there is space on the opposite page for you to make notes.

MONTHS

Your cycle will likely overlap over 2 months. For instance, if your period starts on the 14th January, your cycle months will be: JAN/FEB.

DAYS

Day 1 is the first full day of bleeding. If you begin spotting at 3pm on Tuesday 14th January, your Day 1 will be Wednesday 15th January. In the outer pink rim of your chart find 'day 1' and your entry in there should therefore be: 15.01. If you wish, you can now enter the dates around your entire monthly chart (see example).

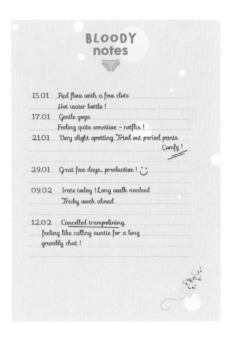

FLOW

The white circle around the edge of the chart has 3 droplets of blood. Colour these drops in according to the quantity of blood you are losing each day.

🌢 🌢 🌢 3 drops = heavy 🌢 🌢 2 drops = medium 🌢 1 = light.

MOON

At the bottom of the page are symbols for each phase of the moon that can be added to the outer red rim of the chart. Look at the lunar calendar and if, for instance, the full moon is on the 11th February, an empty circle can be added to that day.

MONTHS : _____

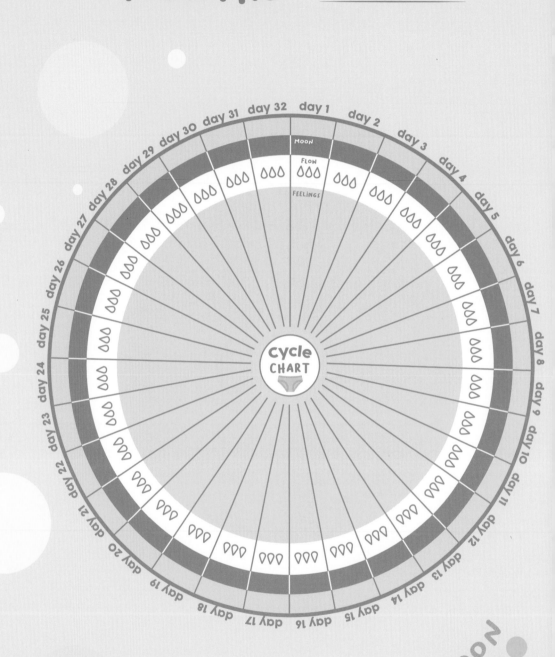

BLOODY notes

MONTHS : _____

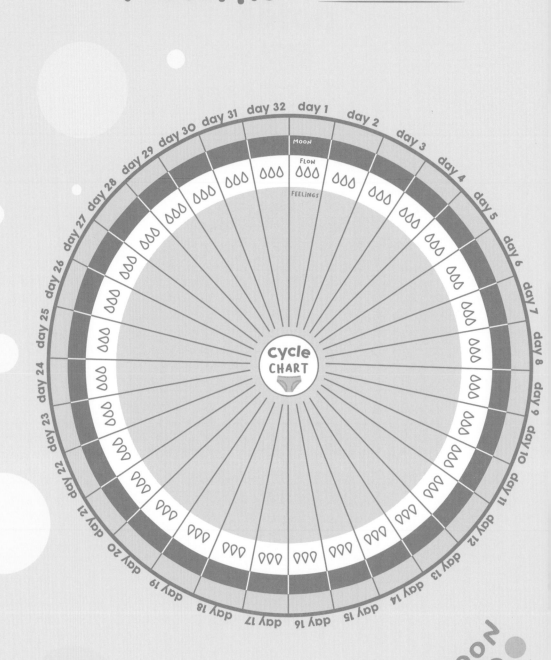

MOON

FULL
WANING
WAXING
NEW

BLOODY
notes

_____

_____

_____

_____

_____

_____

_____

_____

_____

_____

_____

_____

_____

_____

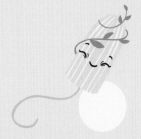

MONTHS : _____

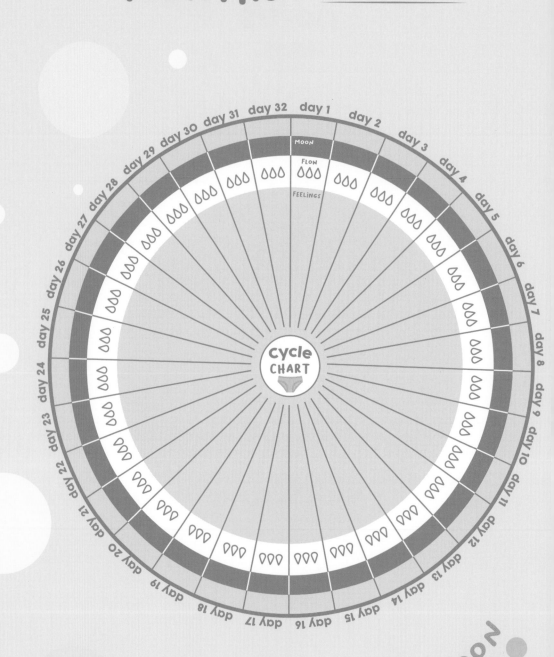

BLOODY
notes

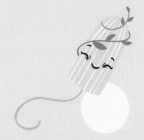

MONTHS : _____

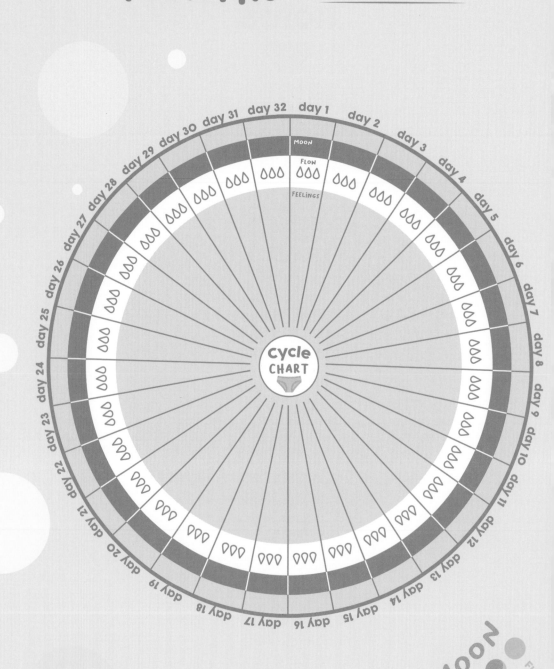

cycle CHART

MOON
FLOW
FEELINGS

day 1 day 2 day 3 day 4 day 5 day 6 day 7 day 8 day 9 day 10 day 11 day 12 day 13 day 14 day 15 day 16 day 17 day 18 day 19 day 20 day 21 day 22 day 23 day 24 day 25 day 26 day 27 day 28 day 29 day 30 day 31 day 32

MOON
Full
Waning
Waxing
New

BLOODY
notes

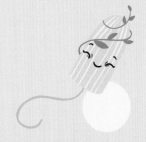

MONTHS : _____

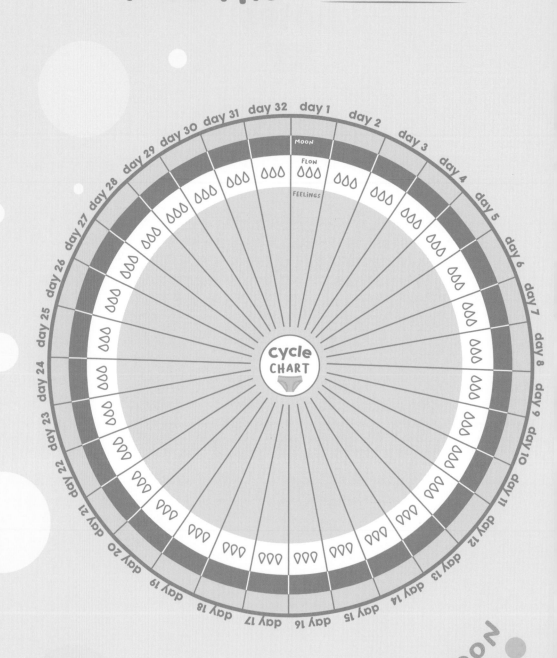

BLOODY notes

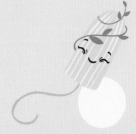

MONTHS : _____

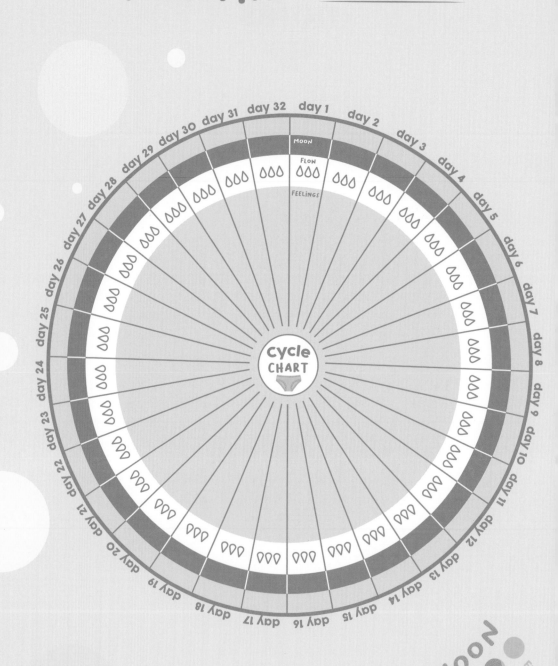

BLOODY
notes

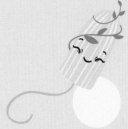

MONTHS : _____

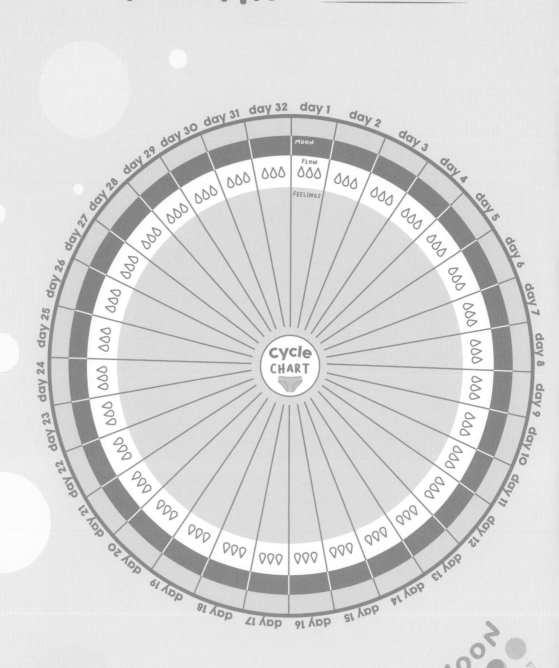

BLOODY
notes

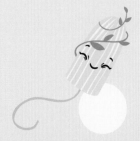

MONTHS : _____

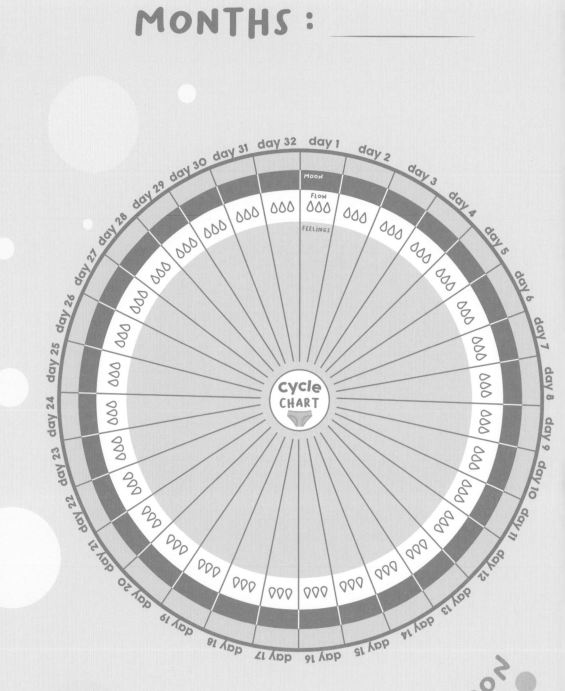

MOON

FLOW

FEELINGS

cycle CHART

day 32 day 1 day 2 day 3 day 4 day 5 day 6 day 7 day 8 day 9 day 10 day 11 day 12 day 13 day 14 day 15 day 16 day 17 day 18 day 19 day 20 day 21 day 22 day 23 day 24 day 25 day 26 day 27 day 28 day 29 day 30 day 31

MOON

Full

Waning

Waxing

New

BLOODY notes

MONTHS : _____

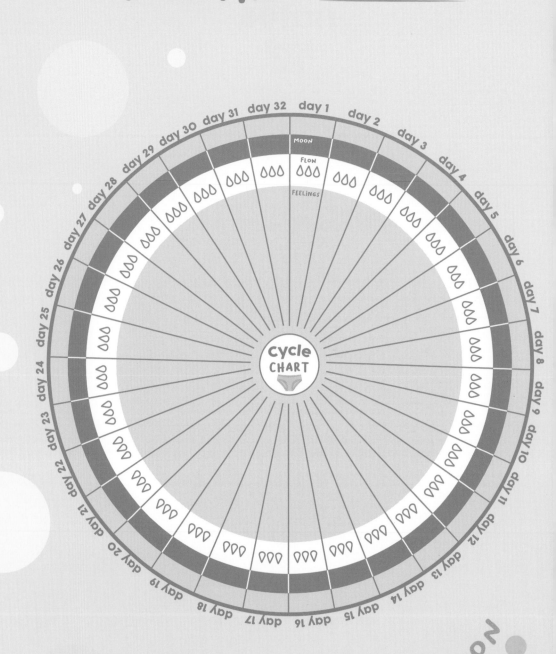

day 32 · day 1 · day 2 · day 3 · day 4 · day 5 · day 6 · day 7 · day 8 · day 9 · day 10 · day 11 · day 12 · day 13 · day 14 · day 15 · day 16 · day 17 · day 18 · day 19 · day 20 · day 21 · day 22 · day 23 · day 24 · day 25 · day 26 · day 27 · day 28 · day 29 · day 30 · day 31

MOON
FLOW
FEELINGS

cycle
CHART

MOON
Full
Waning
Waxing
New

BLOODY
notes

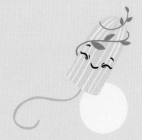

MONTHS : _____

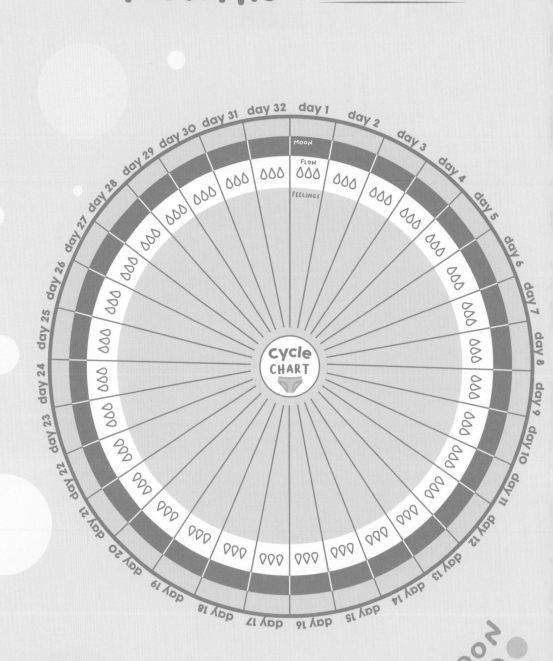

BLOODY notes

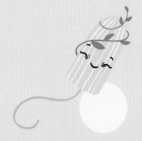

MONTHS : _____

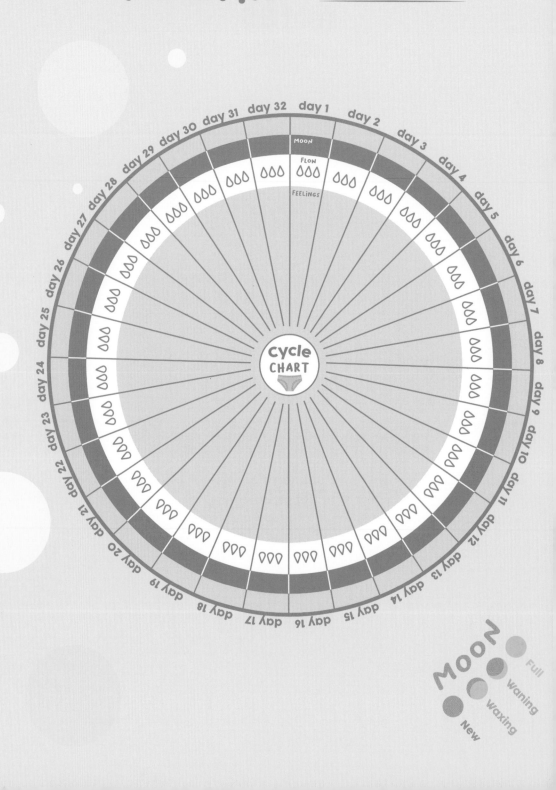

BLOODY
notes

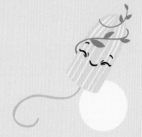

MONTHS : _____

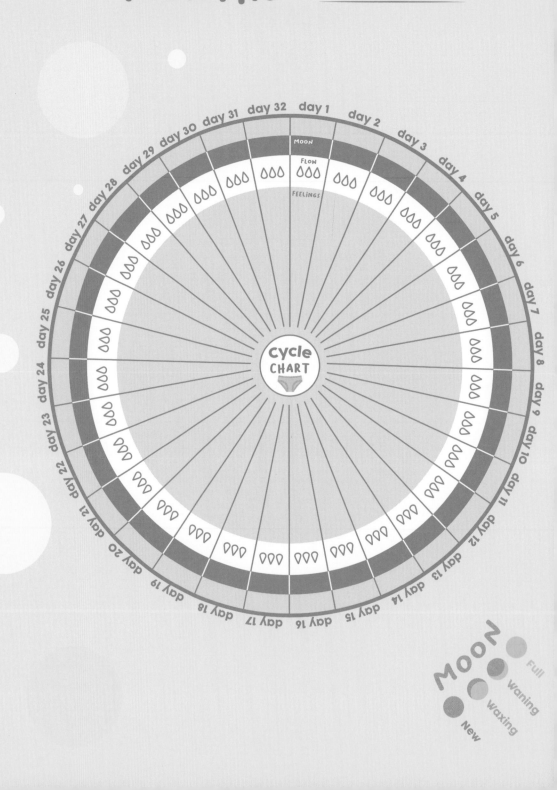

BLOODY
notes

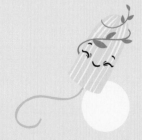

MONTHS : _____

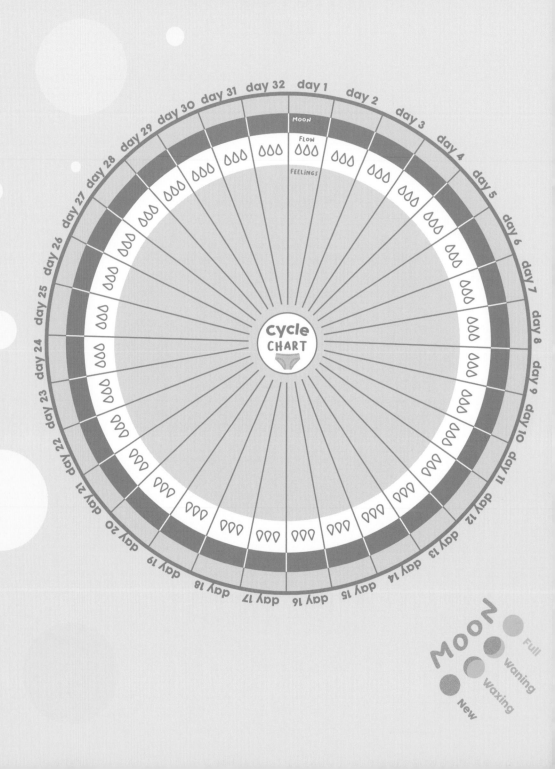

MOON

FLOW

FEELINGS

day 31 day 32 day 1 day 2 day 3 day 30 day 29 day 28 day 27 day 26 day 25 day 24 day 23 day 22 day 21 day 20 day 19 day 18 day 17 day 16 day 15 day 14 day 13 day 12 day 11 day 10 day 9 day 8 day 7 day 6 day 5 day 4

cycle CHART

MOON

Full
Waning
Waxing
New

BLOODY notes

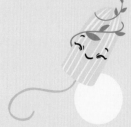

MONTHS : _____

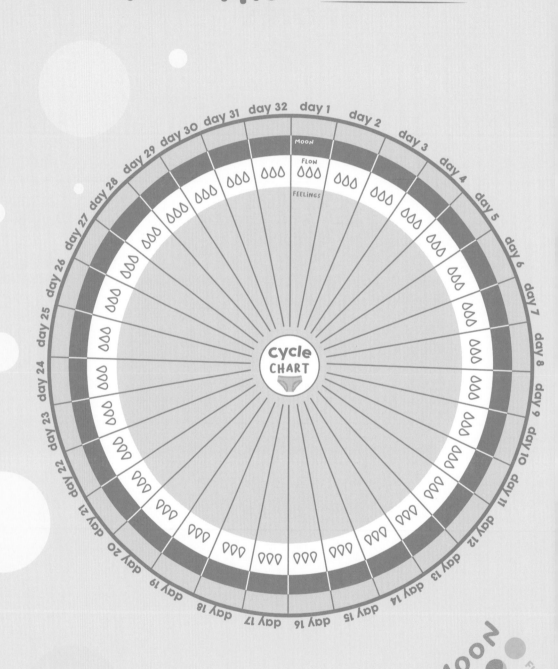

MOON

Full
Waning
Waxing
New

BLOODY notes

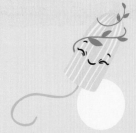

MONTHS : _____

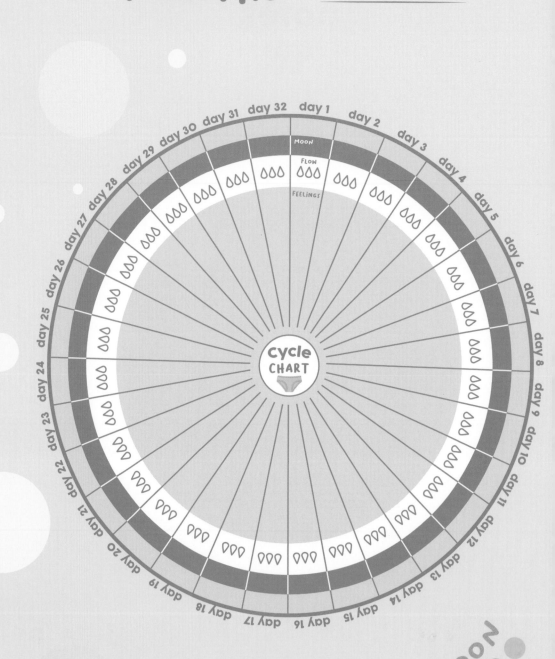

BLOODY
notes

_____

_____

_____

_____

_____

_____

_____

_____

_____

_____

_____

_____

_____

_____

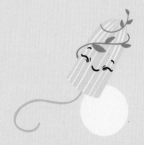

MONTHS : _____

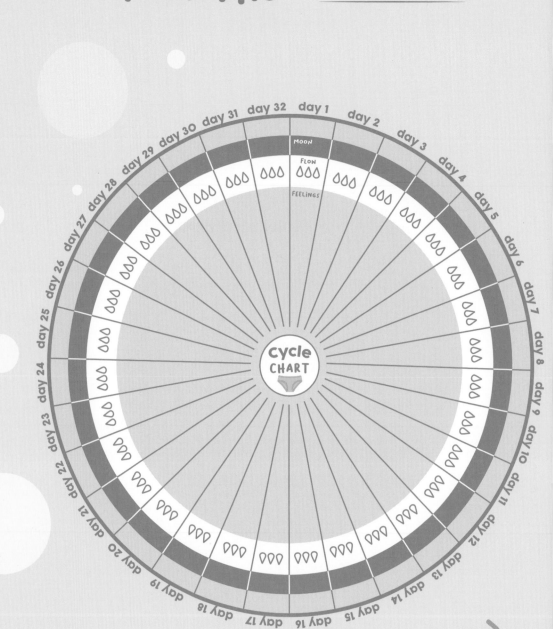

BLOODY
notes

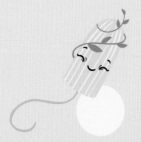

MONTHS : _____

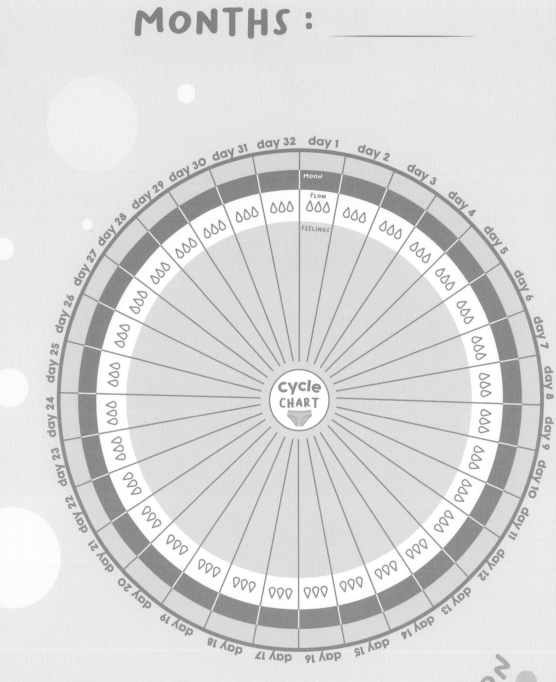

BLOODY
notes

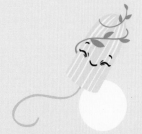

MONTHS : _____

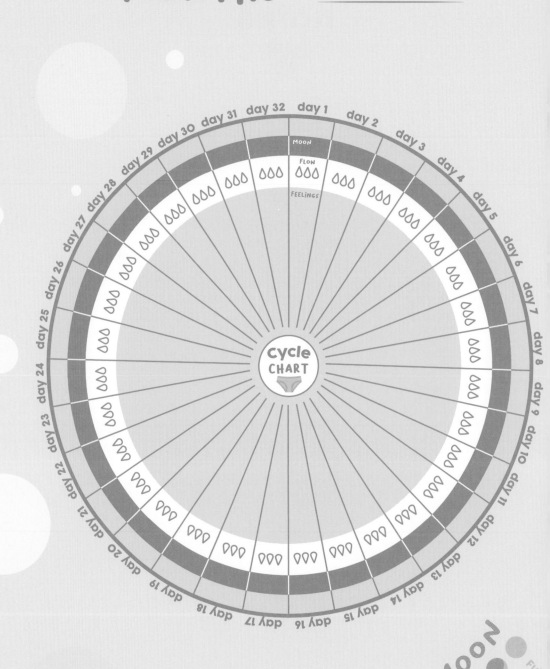

day 32 day 1 day 2 day 3 day 4 day 5 day 6 day 7 day 8 day 9 day 10 day 11 day 12 day 13 day 14 day 15 day 16 day 17 day 18 day 19 day 20 day 21 day 22 day 23 day 24 day 25 day 26 day 27 day 28 day 29 day 30 day 31

MOON
FLOW
FEELINGS

cycle
CHART

MOON
Full
Waning
Waxing
New

BLOODY notes

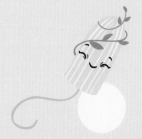

MONTHS : _____

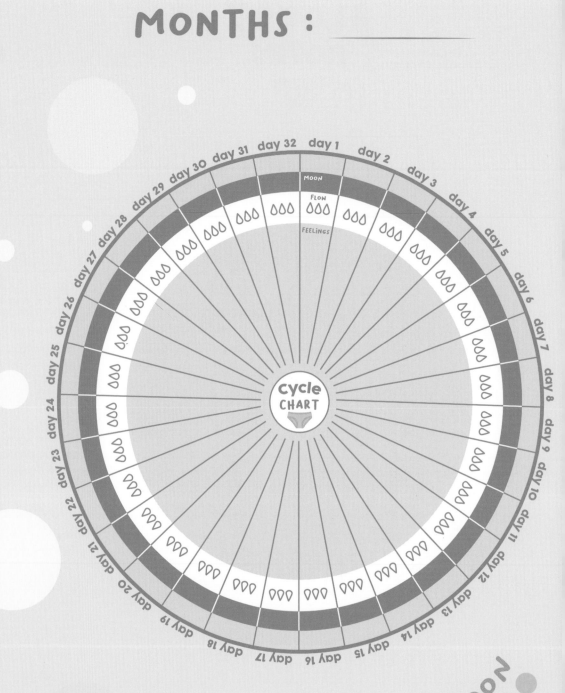

BLOODY notes

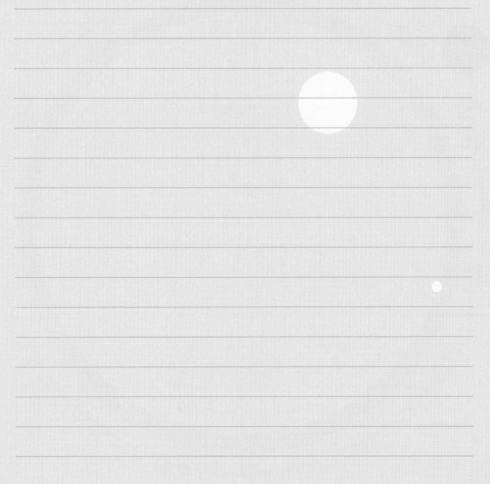

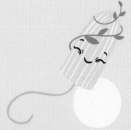

MONTHS : _____

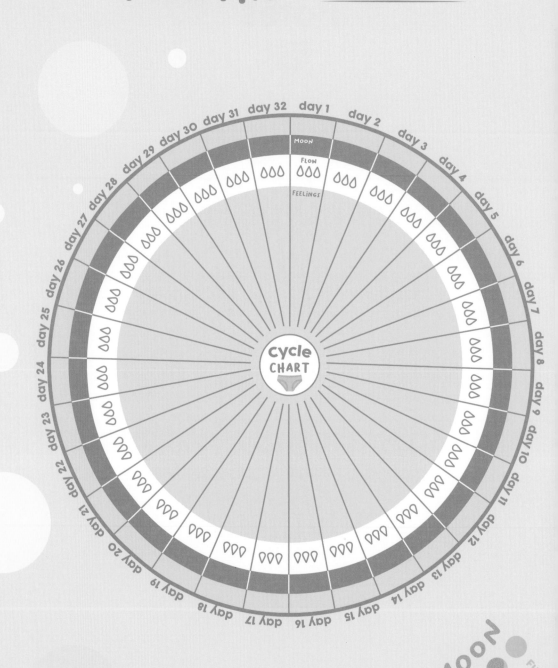

BLOODY notes

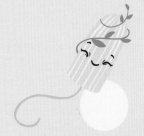

MONTHS : _____

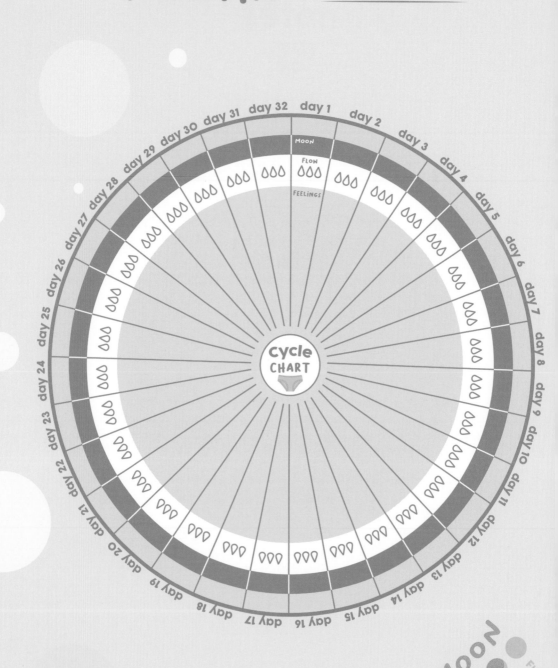

BLOODY
notes

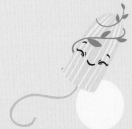

MONTHS : _____

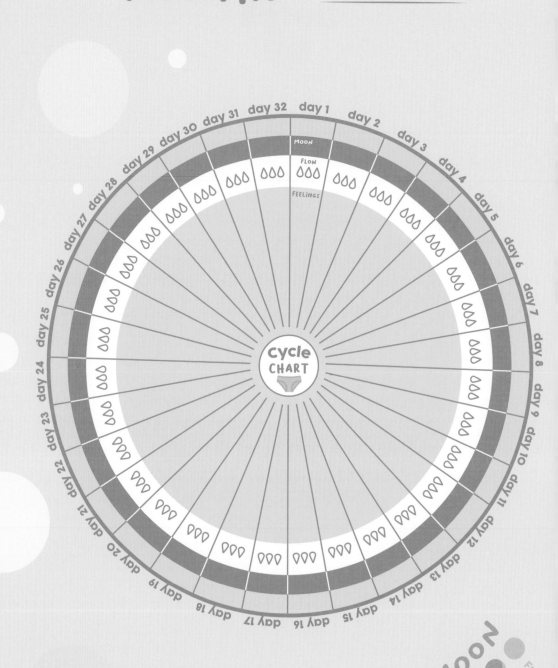

BLOODY
notes

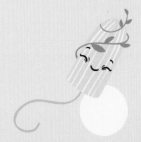

MONTHS : _____

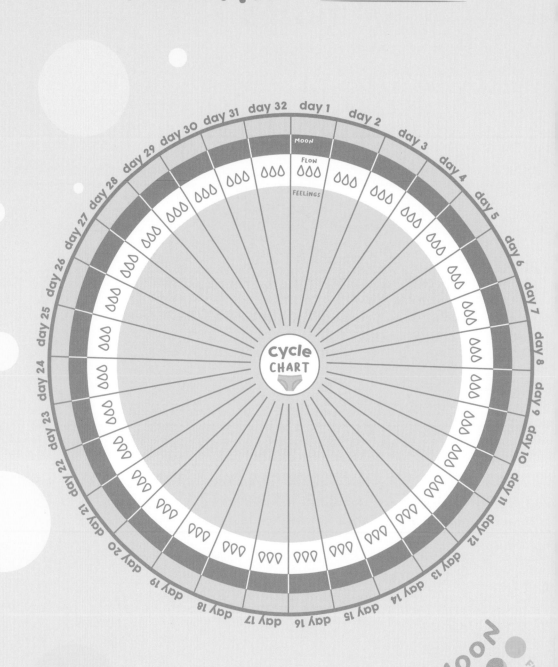

BLOODY
notes

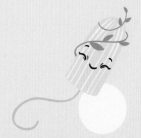

MONTHS : _____

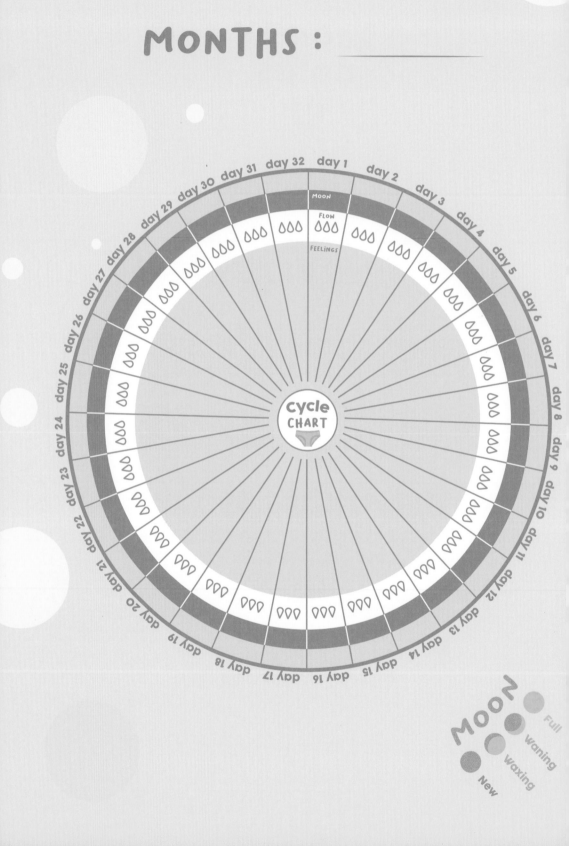

BLOODY
notes

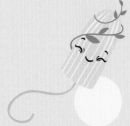

Periods of the year

MONTH OF THE YEAR ....

DAY OF THE MONTH												
1												
2												
3												
4												
5												
6												
7												
8												
9												
10												
11												
12												
13												
14												
15												
16												
17												
18												
19												
20												
21												
22												
23												
24												
25												
26												
27												
28												
29												
30												
31												

Periods of the year

1											
2											
3											
4											
5											
6											
7											
8											
9											
10											
11											
12											
13											
14											
15											
16											
17											
18											
19											
20											
21											
22											
23											
24											
25											
26											
27											
28											
29											
30											
31											

DAY OF THE MONTH

2021 LUNAR CHART

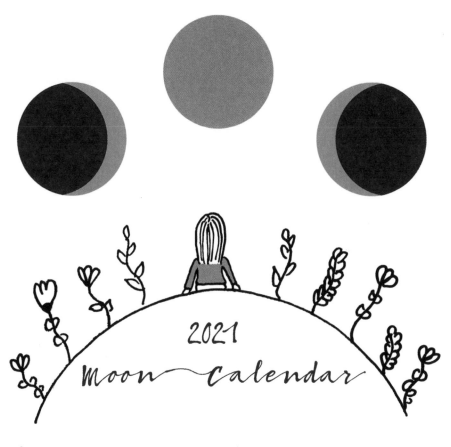

Jan	6	12	20	28		Jul	1	9	17	23	31	
Feb	4	11	19	27		Aug	8	15	22	30		
Mar	5	13	21	28		Sep	6	13	20	28		
Apr	4	11	19	26		Oct	6	12	20	28		
May	3	11	19	26		Nov	4	11	19	27		
Jun	1	10	17	24		Dec	3	10	18	26		

UTERINE REPRODUCTIVE SYSTEM QUIZ

Place the words below to label the diagram
Answers can be found on page 148

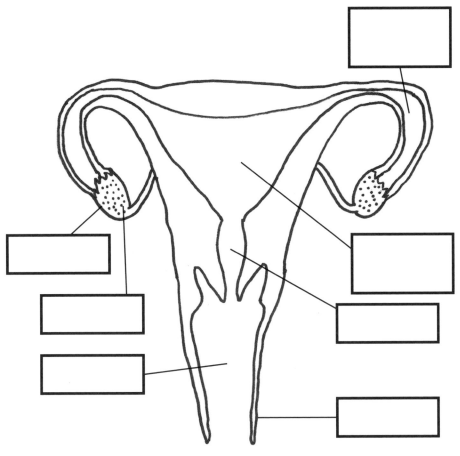

FRONTAL VIEW

Cervix   Ovary   Vagina
Eggs   Fallopian tubes
Labia   Uterus/womb

RE-USABLE PAD TEMPLATE

INSTRUCTIONS

1. Use the black line to cut a template for 2 pieces of soft fabric eg. cotton

2. Use the red line to cut a template for 2 pieces of absorbent fabric eg. towelling or fleece

3. Sew the winged pads together leaving both ends open, and turn inside out

4. Sew along the dotted lines

5. Insert the absorbent layers into the pad, making sure they are even and flat

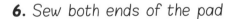

6. Sew both ends of the pad

7. Sew poppers or buttons onto the wings to secure

8. Find some of your favourite fabrics and give as gifts to your friends and family

COLOURING PATTERNS

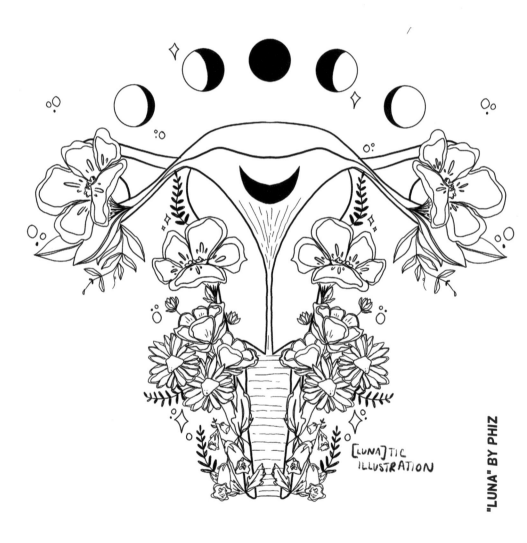

[LUNA]TIC
ILLUSTRATION

"LUNA" BY PHIZ

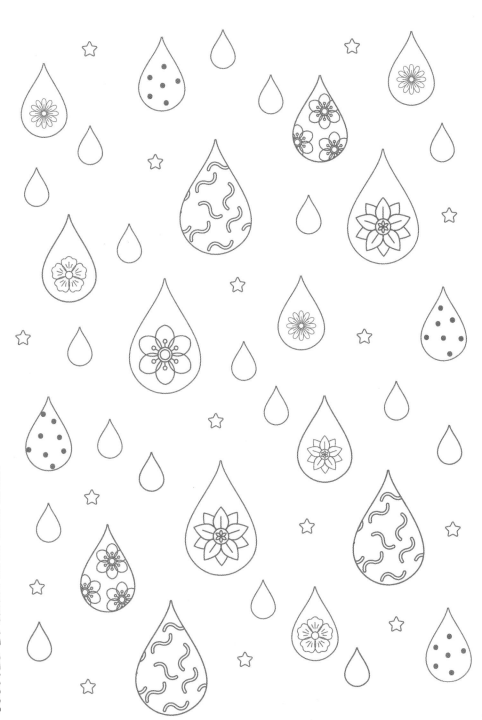

"GOUTTES" BY CAROTTE ET COMPAGNIE

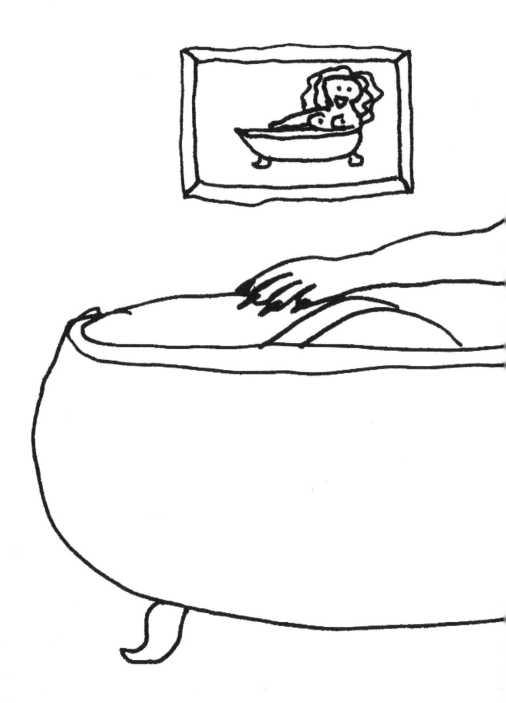

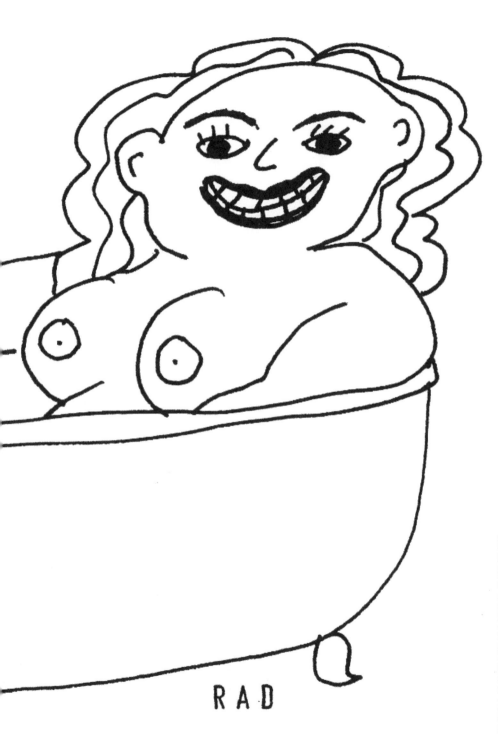

RAD

"BATH BAE" BY RACHEL DUGGAN

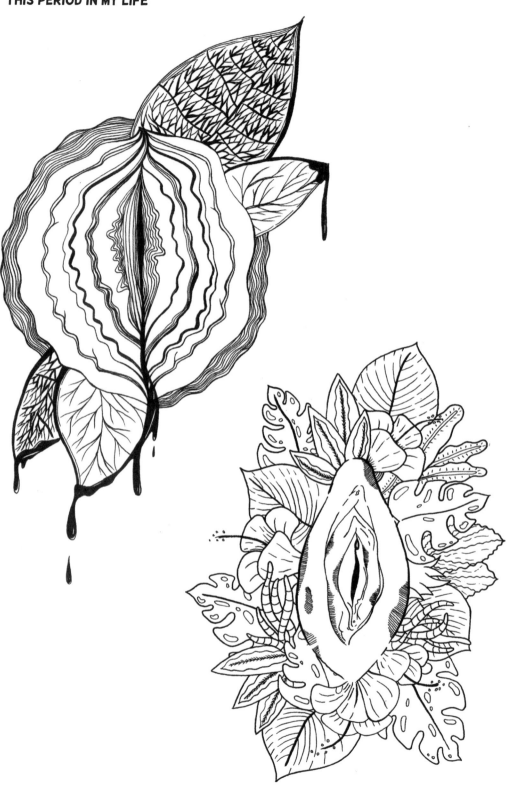

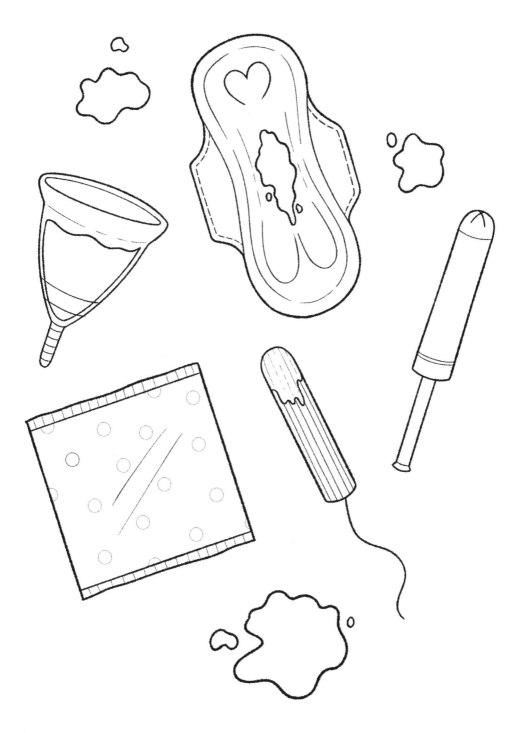

"YOUR BLOODY CHOICE" BY CHARLOTTE WILLCOX

RESOURCES

BOOKS
Period by Natalie Byrne
Period Power by Maisie Hill
Ruby Luna's Curious Journey by Tessa Venuti Sanderson
Vaginas and Periods by Christian Hoeger & Kristen Lilla
My Period Pack Hey Girls (box of cards)

PLACES TO VISIT
The Vagina Museum, London www.vaginamuseum.com

PODCASTS
The Vagina Museum
The Vagina Blog Podcast
Amaze
Dear Teen Girl
Girls 4 Greatness
You Inside Out

WEBSITES
www.amaze.org
www.bettyforschools.co.uk
www.heygirls.co.uk

APPS
Clue
Magic Girl
Period Tracker
Moody
Fitbit
Groove
HH Pro

QUIZ ANSWERS

This is how your labels should have looked for the quiz on page 139

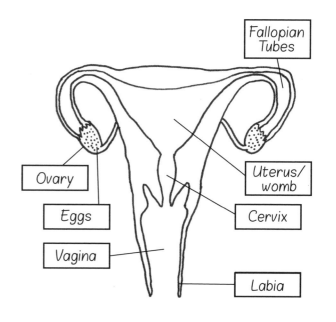

Fallopian Tubes

Ovary

Eggs

Vagina

Uterus/womb

Cervix

Labia

REFERENCES

CHAPTER 1 - FIRST PERIOD
Cultural celebrations of the Menarche taken from this book: Torres-Gomez, J. & Barrow, E.C. (2014) *'Cycling to Grandma's House'*, Lulu Publishing Services.

CHAPTER 5 - TRIAL PERIOD
'First 'fine to flush' wet wipes approved in drive to tackle fatbergs'. Smithers,R. (2019). (Online) Available from: https://theguardian.com/money/2019/feb/26/first-fine-to-flush-wet-wipes-approved-in-drive-to-tackle-fatbers

CHAPTER 6 - YOUR SUSTAINABLE PERIOD
Images from WEN: 'Period action' (Pad): https://www.natracare.com/why-natracare/plastic-free/

'Break Free From Plastic' (Cups): https://www.breakfreefromplastic.org/menstrual-products-report-2019/

CHAPTER 8 - P.E. PERIOD
'Here's why I ran the London Marathon on the first day of my period – and chose not to wear a tampon', Gandhi, K. (2015) (Online). Available from: http://www.independent.co.uk/voices/ comment/heres-why-i-ran-the-london-marathon-on-the-first-day-of-my-period-and-chose-not-to- wear-a-tampon-10455176.html

'Chelsea become first club to tailor training to menstrual cycles'
Rowan,K. (2020), (Online) Available from: https://www.telegraph.co.uk/football/2020/02/13/exclusive-chelsea-become-first-club-tailor-training-menstrual/

'It's because I had my period': swimmer Fu Yuanhui praised for breaking taboo', Phillips, T. (2016) (Online). Available from: https://www.theguardian.com/sport/2016/aug/16/chinese-swimmer-fu-yuanhui-praised-for-breaking-periods-taboo

CHAPTER 13 - PERIODS AROUND THE WORLD
'Cloth, cow dung, cups: how the world's women manage their periods'. Hodal, K. (2019) (Online) Available from: https://www.theguardian.com/global-development/2019/apr/13/cloth-cow-dung-cups-how-the-worlds-women-manage-their-periods

'This Is What Periods Look Like for Women Around The World'. Gil, N. (2019) (Online). Available from: https://www.refinery29.com/en-gb/2019/04/229665/periods-around-the-world-water-aid

REFERENCES

CHAPTER 14 - PERIOD POVERTY
'Break the Barriers: Girls experiences of menstruation in the UK report (2018)', Plan International UK. Pages 11,15,46.

CHAPTER 15 - FREE PERIODS
'The blood drop emoji is appearing on phones and keyboards everywhere. This is why it matters'. Crews,R. (2019) (Online). Available from: https://plan-uk. org/blogs/putting-an-end-to-period-stigma-and-taboo

'The best news in the budget is that tampon tax has been abolished', George,A. (2020) (Online). Available from: https://www.telegraph.co.uk/women/politics/best-news-budget-tampon-tax-has-abolished-period/

'Free period products for all schools and colleges'. Department for Education and Michelle Donelan MP (2020). (Online) Available from: https://www.gov.uk/government/news/free-period-products-for-all-schools-and-colleges

https://en.wikipedia.org/wiki/Amika_George
https://en.wikipedia.org/wiki/Laura_Coryton

'Aldi scraps plastic tampon applicator after campaign'. Menendez,E. (2020). (Online) Available from: https://metro.co.uk/2020/01/23/aldi-scraps-plastic-tampon-applicators-campaign-12109420/

'New York just made menstrual history', McConnell,J. (2019). (Online). Available from: https://msmagazine.com/2019/07/05/new-york-just-made-menstrual-history/

TAKE ACTION www.citytosea.org.uk/plasticfreeperiods/rethink-periods/

CHAPTER 16 - PERIODS IN HISTORY
https://en.wikipedia.org/wiki/Feminine_hygiene#cite_note-:6-38
'Flow: the cultural story of menstruation (2009) Stein, E. (2009), New York: St Martin's Griffin
https://www.bloodandmilk.com/brief-history-of-period-products/

IMAGES:
Hoosier Sanitary Belt: https://de.wikipedia.org/wiki/Monatshygiene
1800s image: http://susannaives.com/wordpress/2015/09/tidbits-on-mid-victorian-era-menstrual-hygiene/
Tampon: http://www.mum.org/Tampaxpatent.htm

ACKNOWLEDGEMENTS

FEATURED ARTISTS
The artists featured in this book have all kindly donated their artwork for the worthy cause of removing stigmas and taboos around periods. Check them out on Instagram!

🩸 **Alex Uxbridge** is an artist inspired by poetry and song, and by his upbringing which provide him with endlessly renewable scope for his imagination. Alex has exhibited numerous one man shows throughout London and the UK. @alexuxbridge

🩸 **Amelia Eve** is an animator, illustrator and fellow menstruator. Her work aims to encourage people to talk about their periods and make friends with 'mother nature', because sometimes you just have to look your period in the eye and say 'we're in it together'. @ameliagraceve

🩸 **April Davis** has been featured in magazines, on podcasts, and on stage, sharing her wisdom, humor and knowledge as the creator of The Vagina Blog and The Vagina Blog Podcast. Her passion and drive have created an entire community around female body health, as she empowers women and vagina owners to love themselves. Web: thevaginablog.com @thevaginablog

🩸 **Charlotte Heillette** (Carotte et Compagnie) is a freelance illustrator and graphic designer. She is inspired by children, stationery, pattern, travel, beautiful books and design generally to bring some air and positivity into our world. @carotteetcompagnie_design

🩸 **Charlotte Willcox** is a freelance illustrator and designer based in the UK. She's a graduate from the University of Southampton with a Bachelor's degree in Graphic Arts. Charlotte is a passionate feminist who enjoys tackling the taboo, and focuses her work on issues such as women's rights, body confidence, politics, the LGBTQ+ community and social issues. www.charlotteillustrates.com @charlotte.illustrates

🩸 **Crystal Kennings** is a menstrual wellness advocate, passionate about breaking the stigma of menstruation through education. @crystalkennings

🩸 **Dhillon Kaur** is an artist and activist currently studying art and design at college in Swansea. She uses her work to create bright and striking imagery which often tackles issues such as body image and period stigma. @dhillonkaurart

ACKNOWLEDGEMENTS

🔹 **Ditti Magyar** is from Hungary but living in California, USA. She is a watercolour and digital artist. Her inspiration comes from the small beauties of life, to encourage us to live in sync with Mama Nature. @BrownBudapest

🔹 **Hannah Phizaclea** is a queer artist and 3D designer based in London. Her illustrations focus on mental health, feminism and queerness. She tries to deal with the big issues through flowers and magic. www.linktr.ee/lunaticillustrations @lunaticillustration

🔹 **Hazel Mead** is a freelance illustrator whose work delves into the depths of taboo and challenges societal norms with a cute playful style often juxtaposed with a satirical, 'bitey' tone. Her work covers a wide range of topics including periods, female masturbation, body image, mental health and the patriarchy. www.hazelmead.com @hazel.mead

🔹 **Holly Lehnmann** is an illustrator and designer living in London who says: "Ever since I got my period I've never shied away from talking about it openly with anyone who will listen. I started writing poetic periods in 2019 as a way to make periods fun and to encourage more people to talk openly about their periods. Let's face it we've all got a hilarious period story to tell." @poeticperiods

🔹 **Kat Cass** is a recent graduate from Edinburgh College of Art and is currently a freelance illustrator based in North-West London. She enjoys telling stories that spark conversations by creating visually playful imagery that blend current social issues and pre-existing mythologies to give ideas character. www.katcassart.com @katcassart

🔹 **Krista King** is a registered dietitian nutritionist, integrative and functional certified nutrition practitioner, and holistic health expert specialising in women's health. Through her online practice, Krista provides virtual nutrition coaching, courses and resources to heal your hormones, digestion and anxiety naturally, using a root cause approach. www.composednutrition.com @composednutrition

🔹 **Lisa Joly** is an illustrator born in Paris. After graduating with a Master in French Literature, she settled down in London where she became a French teacher. She completed a short course on illustration at the University of Arts and regularly publishes her illustrations on Instagram. @lescartounesdelisa

ACKNOWLEDGEMENTS

⬧ **Meera Lee Patel** is an artist and writer who believes that anything is possible. She is the author of My Friend Fear: Finding Magic in the Unknown, a beautiful meditation on fear and how it can guide us to incredible change. Find her online at: www.meeralee.com @meeraleepatel

⬧ **Millie Baring** spends her time illustrating and designing, and making wine around the world. Sometimes she combines the elements. When she's not racing around this amazing globe, she is based in London, UK. www.millustrations.co.uk @themillustrator

⬧ **Natalie Byrne** is a Latina illustrator based in London. She studied Graphic Design at Sheffield Hallam University, and found her illustrative voice combining colour and important topics. Natalie's work promotes intersectional feminism and tackles social issues such as sexual assault, mental health and equality. www.nat-b.com @nataliebyrne

⬧ **Rachal Duggan** is an Illustrator based in Milwaukee, WI. Her body of work revolves around body positivity, storytelling, and pop culture observations. Most recently, her passion project has been illustrating user-submitted period stories in an effort to normalise and destigmatise periods www.rachelduggan.com @radillustrates

⬧ **Sara J Beazley** is a printmaker and artist who has over 15 years' experience in her field. Her innovative approach to printmaking combines traditional printing techniques which have been used in art, design, illustration and retail, amongst others. www.sarajbeazley.com @sarajbeazley

⬧ **Sarah Eichart** is 'Die Menstruationsbeauftragte', which translates as 'the commissioner of menstruation'. She is a German illustrator who wants to change the world and break the taboo around menstruation with her art. www.die-menstruationsbeauftragte.de/mein-blog @diemenstruationsbeauftragte

⬧ **Vanessa Chau** passionately advocates for mental health. She guides you to your own path of self-development by sharing with you the tips, exercises and information that she discovered through her own journey. She is that sister you can hang out with and just talk to about anything and everything under the sun! @theself_carekit

ACKNOWLEDGEMENTS

⬥ At Woman Kind, Leora Leboff and Kate Codrington offer online and in person retreats for those wanting to develop more kindness in their lives. With more than 50 years of experience between them, they have developed unique practices that give an embodied sense of cyclical wisdom so that life can be lived with greater authenticity, creativity and self-kindness. www.woman-kind.co.uk

Thank you to the following organisations for their contributions, images and support!

⬥ City to Sea - citytosea.org.uk
⬥ Period Proof - periodproof.co/
⬥ Plan International UK - plan-uk.org
⬥ Natracare - natracare.com
⬥ Women's Environmental Network - wen.org.uk

 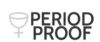 natracare

ACKNOWLEDGEMENTS

WITH THANKS TO...

I'm not sure this book would have left my laptop had it not been for your reaction, Elise, to the news that I was writing a book: "What?! You mean, like, a real book?" Thank you for pushing me to complete it. Every word has been written with you and your sisters in mind. If you, Uma or Lucille even read just one page of this, it will have been worthwhile. Mes bisounours je vous adore!

Gerry, merci for always believing in me, and filling my cup every single day. Legend.

To my parents, Goo, the ultimate Mother Nature, and Nonno the ultimate 'Pacha', thank you for your support, love, warmth and unconditional everything... Jackie, I think your first tampon experience pretty much sums up our sisterhood: close and open! Love ya.

Thank you to Stuart for being a rock star of a designer, putting up with all my late additions and not shying away from blood, and to Lisa, my hawk-eye editor.

Thank you to all the amazing artists and organisations who have donated their images and graphics to the book, and who continue to do astounding work to ditch the bad blood. Forever grateful to you – you are all bloody brilliant.

AUTHOR INFORMATION

Saskia Boujo is a relationship and sex educator who has been teaching young people for almost 20 years. This Period in My Life is her first book, inspired by her own struggles to conceive. Saskia suffered from endometriosis, a debilitating condition that caused her infertility, and she believes that better education around menstruation could have potentially helped her avoid infertility. This, her 3 young children, and the many young people she meets in the classroom, eventually became the inspiration for the book. She continues to proudly fly the fertility flag, though her work educating young people is now her main occupation.

NOTES

NOTES

NOTES

NOTES

NOTES

NOTES

NOTES

NOTES

NOTES

NOTES

NOTES